Your Beautiful Body °

By Othon Molina Ph.D c LMT

The purpose of this book is to assist you in knowing more about your body, how to help yourself and your family, assist in it's healing and improve the quality of your life. For therapists, trainers, coaches or athletes this book will be valuable in its tools and diagnostics of over thirty years experience. Especially for the athlete a valuable tool for improving the functioning of your body, and it's recovery as well.

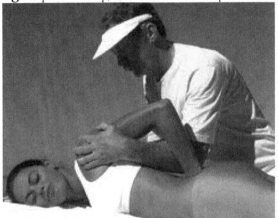

Great pictures are by° Sunstar others by Othon Molina

Othon in Hawaii: "I recommend this book to every serious massage therapist, trainer, coach or interested athlete that wants to understand the mechanical function of "YOUR BEAUTIFUL BODY.""

I want to thank Sunstar for his fantastic pictures and all his support and encouragement, also all the models for letting me massage you and helping with this project. Wana'ao' Watson Eldridge, Leilani Peña, Jennifer Tamaki, Morgan and Vesha. Stay tuned for more books next is "Better back book" following that will be "The Molina Method complete book of training"

Othon Molina has a vast wealth of experience and knowledge to share in his new book. I have known and watched Othon for thirty years expand and explore the very nature of our body's relationship to gravity, stress, sports, relationships, nutrition and the whirling mysteries of thoughts and feelings. He has demonstrated the capacity to introduce brilliant styles and techniques to the realm of "Body Work" both clinically and as a persistent researcher. Othon is continuously exploring the infinite cosmos of human anatomy and physiology. Othon walks his teachings and offers his practical wisdom to those of us eager to learn more of healing to help those we love. Whether you are new to the path of healing and "Body Work" or well down the road you will be rewarded with hands on techniques to help others immediately.

Bruce A. Parker D.C.
Malibu Health and Rehabilitation
Malibu, Ca.

Order this book online at www.trafford.com
or email orders@trafford.com

Most Trafford titles are also available at major online book retailers.

Print information available on the last page.

isbn: 978-1-4120-4869-9 (sc)
isbn: 978-1-4907-6857-1 (e)

Trafford rev. 02/22/2019

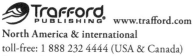 www.trafford.com

North America & international
toll-free: 1 888 232 4444 (USA & Canada)
fax: 812 355 4082

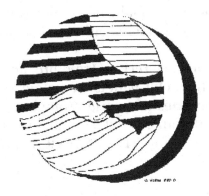

A short summary to get you started on some of the deep discoveries of the last century:

In the last thirty years we have had a renaissance of health and wellness. Our generation is very much going to change the habits of our fathers through the use of massage as well as total fitness programs. We are also in a period of spiritual renewal, and much of what we know as science is crossing over into spiritual understanding.

In ancient times philosophers such as Permideus, Aristotle, and Socrates closely observed Nature, trying to understand her laws and how the universe works. More recently, in the last century scientists like Newton, Planck, and Einstein through their studies of physics continued to attempt to understand the nature of the universe and its laws. Some say that these same laws apply to the nature of human consciousness, that both the physics of our universe and the workings of our consciousness must obey the same laws, and many say these two are actually one and the same. Singularity right!

When Einstein first talked about the universe not having fixed laws, and thereby taking Newtonian physics to a new level, the scientists of the time asked that if the universe is moving, expanding and not fixed, how could we know anything? If it's always moving and expanding, there must be one thing that is a fixed point for us to know or study it.

Einstein responded with one of the most powerful statements of his career: "To know the universe you must pick a fixed point, and that is you! Once you do, you can understand the universe in relation to that fixed point. Then, getting together with another person or another point of view, sharing your information, you now know the universe from two points of view, and so on."

Oh my, that means, in a sense, we have to get together to know everything -- kind of a get-along-with-each-other philosophy -- I like it. Working for peace was one way Einstein directly applied his beliefs. Many people say that he was not a religious person; however, I'm not sure what religion they were referring to.

For those of us non-scientists, this means that we can only know the universe or life from our individual points of view. Of course, the catch to this is that you must know WHO YOU ARE and that may sound redundant. You may say "of course I know who I am!" but knowing who you are also involves knowing clearly what you want from life, without any doubts.

Any un-clarity surrounding these two main principles translates to the universe as un-clarity, and so then you don't truly understand either the universe around you or your life.

What we think is what we are, what we receive from life, and from the universe around us. In other words, it's all our creation. Our beliefs create our reality; our reality creates what we perceive; what we perceive creates the world around us, including our body, which we then "embody" into our selves. It is an eternal loop, and we are the center of our universe. Without us at the center there is nothing. THE UNIVERSE, LIKE LIFE, IS WHAT WE MAKE IT!

There is "a new kid on the block" and I have had the pleasure to take a couple of workshops with him. I've recently completed reading his new paper entitle "A Scaling Law for Organized Matter in the Universe and a New View of Unification." This young man, with Elizabeth Rauscher, has written the law that Einstein spent the last twenty years of his life trying to work out, "The Unified Field Theory."

There is so much within this information that applies to science, astronomy, and physics, but more importantly, to how we live our lives. This is the most important aspect of all this new information. Well, it is for me, and I think it is just as much so for everyone who questions the usefulness of all this knowledge and physics, and wonders "what does this all mean to me in my every day life?"

What it means, of course, is that we are each ultimately responsible for our own life and the universe around us. Some people agree, and then say in the same sentence "yes, I'm responsible for everything in my life, well, everything that is, except the time that tourist ran into my car." Well, it doesn't quite work that way -- it's all or nothing.

It presents us with a host of questions: If I create my entire universe, then do I create my own pain and my own illness? And what about disease: Is there being in-balance in the universe, and can I ever be out of balance? Is there death?

What about a paradox -- can there be paradoxes in the universe? ... (Well, I don't think so.) And what is pain? That is the question that is the focus of this book.

This book is dedicated to Rene Teresa Molina who taught me the power of love, and the strength that comes with the faith in life. To our son Othon Wai'ao lani Molina who has taught me about being a father and my daughter Gabriella Lehua Molina who is my greatest love and both who continually awaken me to the beauty and richness of life.

ACKNOWLEDGEMENTS:

To the consummate student in all of us, who seeks knowledge and better ways to apply it. Let us continually cultivate wisdom of this amazing body. I want to thank my students who always keep pushing me for greater clarity and detail. And to all the doctors and sports medicine physicians whom I have known over the years that have been an inspiration to me. They have allowed me to learn from their vast knowledge and at a very practical level, right there "in the trenches." We all need to realize one thing: The human body is too vast a creation for any one person to know all. That's why we need to work together, those of us who work in the health field as professionals as well as all human beings sharing this planet and this reality.

My thanks to all my friends who keep me real, and to my colleagues who have shared their knowledge, and to the constant focus of our students.

I owe my knowledge of sports medicine to:

Most of all, to my friend, Bernard Portner, M.D., who allowed me to work in his clinic for three intense and solid years. He taught me more about the back and neck during that time, compared to twenty years of doing therapy and learning on my own and with other doctors. And not just about the back, as we worked with the whole body, specializing in back, neck, and sports injuries. During that time we handled pretty much every type of injury you have ever seen. This clinic setting was a very intense, acute injury environment; I call it "training in the trenches."

John Tie, D.C., who gave me my first start in the business of health after pestering him for weeks to give me a job. His partner at the time, Leroy Perry, D.C., inspired me to work with athletes as his specialty in Kinesiology was applied to many of the top athletes.

Bernard Jensen, D.C., a dear friend and one of my first real teachers in iridology as well as in nutrition.

For a new look at the world through my friend, Christian Smidtt, N.D.(in memory of), & Richard Rovin, N.D., both good friends who showed me how to use the many holistic tools available to help people at a very practical level in an everyday practice.

Evarts Loomis, M.D., "the father of holistic medicine" who showed me the ancient ways of natural health systems of organic foods, meditation, and exercise, and how blending these with the new technologies was the best way of healing the whole person.

Terry Albriton, a world champ and the strength coach for the University of Hawaii at Manoa, for his work and dedication to training.

And to the many other doctors with whom I studied and worked during the past thirty years, far too many to mention all of them here. Thank you all.

Most of all, to my best friends since 1976 and fellow therapists, Bruce Parker, D.C., and Barry Nutter, D.C., who have inspired me constantly and have served as sounding boards for my crazy ideas and therapy systems.

There are many, many more to whom I owe thanks. Perhaps one of the last I mention here is my very first teacher, Evaristo Madero, a Yaqui Indian from Mexico whom I had the pleasure to know, and who took me from being an architect graduate student to becoming a healer. Through the study of herbs and with natural manual healing methods he was one of the last of the "Curanderos." Curanderos are holistic healers using herbs, nutrition or chemistry, and manipulations or massage in healing the mind and spirit. Although I was only able to be with Everisto Madero for six months, he taught me almost daily. He got me in touch with what my life was to be about. My calling was as a healer, and my studies in architecture served me as a foundation and created understanding of the structure, balance, and mechanics of the human body.

Look for my future books: Total Training Manual and Molina Body Alignment as well as Curanderos, The Last of the Ancient Healers of Mexico.

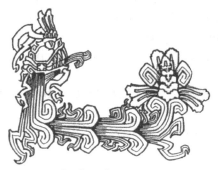

Drawing by Johnny Congas

Introduction

What is this body? Who made it? And how does it all work? What a miracle. I have always wondered where the manual for this body ended up. Everything else on this planet now comes with a guidebook or detailed manual, even your toaster. So where is the manual to the world's most complicated mechanical wonder ever – the human body?

Why are we not taught how the body works? I mean, how it really works at a practical level, how the different parts work in unison, and what all the organs do, in simple language that we can understand or even apply to our lives. It seems that some of the information is available only if you choose medicine as a career. We get a little information in grammar school, some in high school, some in college, and if we're lucky, some of it even sticks. But are we really taught how the body works?

More importantly, why aren't we taught how to tune it up, or, God forbid, how to fix it? Are we really taught how to keep our bodies in good running condition? I don't really think so, at least not the majority of us. If you're a doctor, well, then you know most everything about the body -- unless you're a podiatrist, and then you concentrate your expertise on feet. Or if you're a dermatologist, well, then you focus your career on the skin. Of course, they do teach you about the whole body in medical school but once your specialty is chosen, it takes precedence.

On the subject of medical expertise, many of my doctor friends confirm that if you don't use it, you lose it. I haven't met a doctor yet who knew everything about all areas, and how could we expect them to! There is too much to know. That's why we have specialists now. Don't get me wrong, I totally support and admire the commitment that doctors make.
I may not be a doctor but I have worked and have the experience of thirty years of practice to really start to understand the human body. This body of ours represents a huge body of knowledge, and we are constantly learning new things.

We could spend a lifetime studying the human body and never learn all there is to know about it. Some doctors, naturopaths, chiropractors, and manual therapist and trainers like me have spent our whole lives studying the body, and the more we study, the more there is to learn. It's truly a miracle --how could anyone not believe in God when one considers the miracle of the human body. This is my main reason for saying that we need to work together synergistically, as Bucky Fuller said, for then we have all the systems working together. It all has to work together much as we as humans need to share the same planet.

Where does someone begin to write a book about the overwhelming human body? I've been writing this book for over 20 years and I couldn't get myself to complete it for so long, mainly because the subject is so huge and the details so staggering in quantity.

There are thousands of books on the body, anatomy, physiology, psychology, sports medicine, training, nutrition, yoga, health, and on and on. Read all you can. I've never heard of a bad book -- well, maybe there's one out there.

I have tried to create a book for the basic person on this planet to gain a better understanding of how this body works and to learn some tools to work with it, or at least to accelerate the natural healing ability of the body.

I have written an owner's manual to accompany the human body; one that I hope will be easy to understand, despite some occasionally intense subject matter. I hope to take you on a journey of your body and lead you as far as you are willing to go into this vast universe of information. If you find anything you don't care to explore or don't want details about, just pass it by. I've tried to keep the book simple, readily understandable, and full of information that you can apply to your own body so you can do something about your own health. Only you can change your body. If you are dedicated and willing to make the effort, you can do it. The books are a series, beginning with this one, and then moving into the training of the body and my specific manual therapy.

We can heal in the most incredible ways with knowledge and some action. I will leave the scientific and medical books to the experts. My purpose is to condense all the information I have learned in the last 33 years into a usable form for everyday use.

I will attempt to put massage, training, nutrition, yoga, stretching and body mechanics into a usable format to allow the reader at least a place to begin.
I hope to share a beam of insight into these marvelous machines we run around in. If you want more, there will be more books in this series, so stay tuned.

Anterior muscles

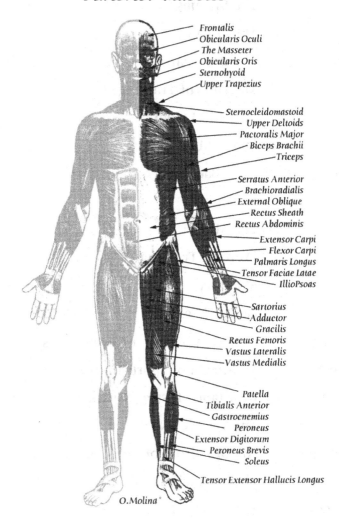

Frontalis
Obicularis Oculi
The Masseter
Obicularis Oris
Sternohyoid
Upper Trapezius

Sternocleidomastoid
Upper Deltoids
Pactoralis Major
Biceps Brachii
Triceps

Serratus Anterior
Brachioradialis
External Oblique
Rectus Sheath
Rectus Abdominis

Extensor Carpi
Flexor Carpi
Palmaris Longus
Tensor Faciae Latae
IllioPsoas

Sartorius
Adductor
Gracilis
Rectus Femoris
Vastus Lateralis
Vastus Medialis

Patella
Tibialis Anterior
Gastrocnemius
Peroneus
Extensor Digitorum
Peroneus Brevis
Soleus

Tensor Extensor Hallucis Longus

O.Molina

Table of Contents

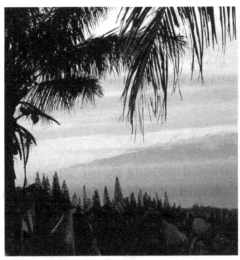

CHAPTER ONE
The Systems

The first and most important aspect of health and the body needs to start with understanding how the systems work and how the individual parts work together. Of course, the body is one whole and very complex organism. It is affected by many aspects of life including the mind and a mental attitude, the structural alignment of the body, what we eat, what we don't eat ... it's very complicated for most of us to really understand. That's why many times we fail to help most people with sickness or pain, because many of us who are health practitioners can't know all aspects of the whole system. And that's why I think it's imperative to learn as much as you can about all aspects, and to experiment with your own body. Once you have some knowledge and find the best system of health and fitness for you, you can apply this knowledge to your own health. Those programs for health can be as different as we humans are individual, and there are far too many variables to list.

The safest as well as the most successful health or athletic development programs rely on science and on a working knowledge of the body, its systems, and the laws of training. Complete training in some way or another involves the interplay of the major systems of the body, the processes, the organs, the muscles, etc. All of these systems will be discussed in some detail throughout the book. It's important that you become familiar with each of these systems if you wish to gain insight about how they synergistically affect your overall health and your specific physical and performance skills. This can be especially important if you are an athlete in training, a manual therapist, a coach or a very active individual.

This manual will talk about training and athletic events, however, our next book, *Total Body Training*, will go into much more detail. It's meant not only for athletes, because as you will see, everyone needs to train in some fashion to stay in shape and achieve their fullest health. This book is designed to teach you an overall understanding of the systems. We will go into more detail about body mechanics as well as injuries, and very detailed information about each muscle. This book is more of a mechanical manual of the body with overviews of the other aspects that contribute to the health of your body.

The Major Systems of the Body

The major systems of the body are the skeletal system, the nervous system, the cardiovascular and respiratory systems, and the metabolic processes, digestion and elimination.

1. The Skeletal System

The bones of the body are designed to hold us up, whether we are sitting or standing. It should take hardly any muscle action to hold the body up. If it does, it is compensating and eventually the stress can create tension and cause the first symptom, aches, or pain. The bones are also designed to protect the internal organs of the thoracic cavity with a cage built up by the ribs and spine. The bones are a source of calcium ions for the blood; the marrow of the bones creates the red blood cells. The bone's weight is about 35% of the total body weight, and along with the teeth, bones are the hardest living tissue in the body, representing our deepest convictions in life. The bones don't actually provide movement; they are the levers by which muscles move the body.

2. The Muscular System

To get a grasp of the scientific approach to fitness conditioning, it's important to understand the muscular system. There are over 400 major skeletal muscles which attach either directly or indirectly to the body's skeletal system. All body movement involves the direct participation of skeletal muscles and movement is always by contraction. Muscles are activated by nerve impulses transmitted from the central nervous system. You possess varying degrees of voluntary and involuntary control over all of these muscles. When the nerve impulse arrives from the brain, the targeted muscle fiber contracts or shortens and brings the origin and insertion (the moving part of the muscle) toward each other. The shortening of the muscle causes the levers of the skeleton to move in a direction relative to where and how the muscle connects to the bone. This is how all movement is produced, and knowing their movement allows us to strengthen that ability by offering resistance in the action of movement.
Part of training is also increasing or improving the ability to use oxygen; this is called aerobic conditioning.

Skeletal muscles have two or more attachments and when they shorten, they apply equal force on the attachments at both ends. The body's movement depends on the stability of each bone and the joint to which it is attached. As a result, the portion that generally moves is the insertion point, usually at the distal attachment, which is located at the farther end from the body midline. We cover levers and movement in greater detail in coming chapters.

As a result of coordinated skeletal muscle contractions made in correct sequence and with adequate force, we are able to talk, walk, run, throw, lift weights, write and make almost any other movement. To improve the body's physical performance in speed, flexibility, strength or muscular endurance, we have to take into consideration all five laws of training. Each of these qualities of fitness requires very specific action to produce improvement.

The need for oxygen is obvious, without it we die. But breathing is not the only thing we need to do to get oxygen into the body. We have to do some sort of aerobic training to really get the health benefits of oxygen penetrating into the deeper tissues. If we become sedentary, the body will start to shut down. But even small amounts of exercise will tell the body we are not a couch potato. Part of training is getting the body to be more effective in using oxygen throughout the tissues and all the way down into the cellular level.

First, in order to improve any physical skill, we must provide the appropriate stress to the muscles in a progressive way. We must establish a base from which to build the body. The theory of adaptability and irritability enables the muscle fiber to adjust to that stress and to strengthen and become more efficient. This all depends on the type of overload stress placed on the body and what you are attempting to do with it.

The type of stress you put on the body will depend on what use you're building towards. (See "specificity" in Chapter Two, The Laws of Training).

For instance, to develop speed, which is a combination of the frequency and force of muscle fiber contraction, both strength and flexibility must improve. We must apply speed-type overload stress. You can't train by running seven-minute miles if you want to compete at four-minute miles or less. This is called specificity of training, and it's the most important theory of athletic development. Remember, in order to increase any specific physical skill, the stress you apply must be appropriate and very specific.

Outside of the purely physical skills, the keys to improving your performance most effectively are as follows:

A. Determine what specific muscles are involved in the actual movement of your desired action, performance skill or sport.

B. Study the actual physical demands on those muscles as well as the cardiovascular needs in a competition situation of your performance skill.

C. Figure out the optimum combination of physical and neurological talents necessary for excellence in that specific skill.

D. Design your training program to duplicate and exaggerate those physical demands as closely as possible in strength, speed, and endurance.

E. Always take into account flexibility and nutrition with all training or health programs. The more accurate your strategy and the safer your training, the more efficiently your target skills will develop, and, consequently, the better results you will get.

3. The Autonomic and Voluntary Nervous Systems

The nervous system is divided into two broad functional categories, one is called autonomic, and the other, voluntary. The autonomic nervous system operates all the subconscious life support functions of the body, per se. This includes actions commonly thought of as ones we have no control over such as the heartbeat, digestion, and arterial action. While it's true that we have little or no conscious control over the heart's functioning, there is plenty of evidence that we can help it work better and stronger. To live longer getting fit is one of the most important facets of life, especially for us baby-boomers. And we all know that the quality of our life is just as important as longevity.

One of the major functions of the voluntary nervous system, on the other hand, is the operation and control of the skeletal muscle system. This system is of primary importance for physical development because we are able to more consciously control many of its functions through action.

All movement requires the direct involvement of the brain and nervous system or it simply will not occur. Without the presence of nerve impulses, muscles don't contract. Without the brain and nervous system, we could not survive. The fact that all movement and "aliveness" is so closely tied to the nervous system and the brain highlights their significance in athletic, health and fitness development.

The mind is the greatest muscle. We have just begun to understand its power; forget about harnessing it, we have a long way to go. Coordination and mental strength are particularly important when you're talking about the speed, agility, strength and finesse needed for fine motor movement. More important are developing the abilities to overcome the mental obstacles we create for ourselves.

Central and Peripheral Nervous Systems

Both nervous systems also have two physical divisions as well. The central nervous system consists of the brain and spinal cord. The peripheral nervous system connects the brain and spinal cord to the rest of the body through its nerves. It's been said that we only use about 10%-20% of the existing voluntary nervous system potential of our brain. It's not, as we have heard, that we only use 10% of the brain, which many people believe. I just would not want to brag about that little fact, anyway. Well, we won't go there now, but see my section on the Mind for more discussion.

The body can handle even the most strenuous of activities with ease when properly trained. The science of all athletic development is slowly unlocking the secrets of how to best develop both body and mind. Your voluntary nervous system ultimately controls how many, how often, and how well these skeletal muscles contract and that relates directly to performance. Imagine what you could physically accomplish if you tripled the function of your voluntary nervous system to 30% or 40% of its capacity. Well, I think we're starting to see that personal development in sports and athletics is all about the nervous system.

Athletes all over the world are breaking records that we thought were unsurpassable. We have high school kids breaking records set just ten or more years ago by Olympic adults. It's amazing where we are taking this body. Research on imagery and mental relaxation in athletics has been out for some time. The mind should be developed along with the rest of the body to get the most out of training, which can open us to many Eastern practices like yoga, tai chi, and the martial arts. They integrate both physical and mental training, and that is the best of both worlds.

4. The Cardiovascular System

These next two sections describe the components of the cardiovascular and respiratory systems, their individual and combined functions, and their relevance to your athletic and fitness conditioning.

A. Heart (Cardio)

The heart is the body's blood pump, a uniquely powerful muscle designed to keep blood circulating constantly throughout the body, all the way down into the molecular level. Because blood is the transport mechanism for oxygen and for the many nutrients that are necessary to sustain life, the ability to move blood quickly and efficiently will determine the amount of physical stress a person can withstand. The heart is the main contributing factor to moving the blood throughout the body. With proper training, you can greatly increase the heart's efficiency. We will go into more detail about strengthening the heart in our training manual and in the aerobic section of this book.

The most important quality that we aim to develop within the heart muscle is cardiac output, which is measured by the volume of blood the heart pumps, and by how fast the heart cleanses that blood, also critical to its performance.

Two factors determine this:

1. Heart Rate = the number of times your heart beats per minute.
2. Volume = the amount of blood that the heart can pump with each beat.

There are many scientifically proven ways to improve both of these functions. All health programs emphasize the need to have a healthy heart, not only for general health but also in relation to the demands of playing or competing in sports.

B. The Vascular System

The vascular system refers to the physical channels through which blood flows. These include the blood vessels or arteries, arterioles, capillaries, venules, and veins. They are categorized by size and function.

1. Size - arteries, which can be quite large, are direct lines from the heart carrying nutrients and oxygen all the way to the capillaries, which are microscopic. These then direct the supply of blood into the cell tissues.

2. Function - function refers to whether they are transport structures for pumping oxygenated blood from the heart to the cells, arteries, arterioles or capillaries, or whether they are returning the waste products (used blood) from the cells to the heart, the venules or veins.

In all, the vascular system is a little like a water pipe system, but in the human body the pipes are flexible and can actively adjust their pressure by expanding or contracting to create the proper blood flow.

Proper exercises can greatly increase the efficiency of this system, ultimately improving the tolerance for increased workloads and greater physical stress, while shortening recuperation time, and best of all, increasing health.

5. The Respiratory System

This system has two primary functions: to load the blood with transportable oxygen, the body's most important nutrient, and to carry away and dispose of carbon dioxide, the cells' main waste product.

There are basically three exchanges of gas within the respiration process: the exchange of gases into and out of the lungs; the exchange of gases between the lungs and blood; the exchange of gases between blood and cells. The two primary gases involved in these processes are oxygen (O_2) and carbon dioxide (CO_2).

The whole purpose of athletic training is to physically strengthen the body and increase its efficiency to both process fuel (nutrients) and to rid itself of toxins. Athletic training is designed to increase the functioning of the body. The role that oxygen plays is the most important, not only in athletic training but also for basic health as well. The more oxygen you can get from the lungs to the tissues, the longer your body can withstand physical stress. It's not just the muscles and cells, but the whole system must become more efficient. We will go into more detail of this subject in the training chapter. Suffice it to say that oxygen plays an all important role in producing the body's main energy fuel source, ATP (adenosine triphosphate).

Athletic training is also designed to improve the body's ability to eliminate carbon dioxide, the primary waste product, from the cells. Your physical fitness depends on the effectiveness of your respiratory system's ability to dispose of CO_2.

Endurance

Endurance is defined as the ability to withstand prolonged physical stress, or to resist fatigue. By cumulatively increasing stress on the body yet remaining aware of the physical structure, endurance can be improved. Physiologists normally classify endurance into two categories: cardiovascular endurance (Wind) and muscle endurance (structural, base or strength). Endurance is largely defined in terms of the efficiency of the cardiovascular and respiratory systems to effectively move oxygen.

After all, these are the systems that provide the oxygen and nutrients (the basic components of ATP-energy production) to the cells and tissues, and rid the body of its waste products on both gross and cellular levels.

6. The Metabolic Process
Energy Production: Its Use and Storage

Metabolism is the process by which the body's tissues produce, store, and retrieve energy. This is a physiological function of vital importance to athletic performance and to life in general. The reasoning is simple: all cells and tissues in the body require energy or else they will cease to function, period.

In relating energy needs to muscles, it is equally as simple. The amount of energy available directly influences the muscles' collective response whether it is a simple everyday task like walking up a flight of stairs, a drawn out test of endurance, or an effort of all out power, as in running up a flight of stairs. (This, of course, also depends on the input of other systems, since all components of the body work together synergistically). The goal in athletic training is to maximize the muscular system's ability to create, use. and store energy, as well as the cardiovascular system to move and cleanse the blood. You can then realize your full athletic potential, according to the energy demands of the particular sport or lifestyle that you desire.

ATP

The predominant energy currency of the body is a substance called ATP or adenosine triphosphate. Simply put, ATP is to your body what gasoline is to a car engine. Although the actual production and storage of ATP is a complex process, I will try to describe it as simply as possible.

ATP is produced from digested foods, usually carbohydrates, which break down into various forms of glucose before reaching the cells. Once the food is in glucose form, it is stored in the cell's mitochondria (power plant) and in other locations of the body such as the liver. We know that there is usually an ample supply of ATP. Glucose is then converted to ATP with the help of oxygen, an all important catalyst throughout the ATP process. Remember, without glucose or oxygen, ATP, the body's basic food, cannot be produced. It is crucial for both the function of the body and for health.

There are three distinct energy production/storage systems that the body uses, and they are classified as being ANAEROBIC (occurring without the presence of oxygen), AEROBIC (occurring with oxygen present), and the Lactic Acid System. Energy for short-strength sports like football comes predominantly from the anaerobic system, and it's important to understand how it operates in order to improve each function. Remember, all training must imitate and exaggerate the method needed for the specific activity.

A. The ATP System (0-30 seconds)

Because football, baseball or soccer (some of us have doubts about this sport being more aerobic) are games of short all-out bursts, usually 10 to 20 seconds of activity followed by rest periods (or semi-rest while still running or moving), the ATP system is the predominant energy system that these sports use. Stored in the mitochondria of each muscle cell are "pools" of ATP for immediate use.

15

The goal of our training program is to make these ATP pools as large as possible, and to develop the capacity to replenish them quickly during the rest phase before they are depleted again. Most sports fit into this category, except for the longer running sports, or long distance swimming, longer triathlons, and some long bicycle events.

B. **The Lactic Acid System** (30 seconds - 3 minutes)

When you deplete your initial stores of ATP through near maximal effort --for most athletes this takes from 30 to 60 seconds -- you move into the Lactic Acid System.

This system is definitely the most painful to develop because the process causes muscular soreness. You have probably run out of this energy and have experienced the phenomenon of "hitting the wall." Once you deplete those initial pools of ATP, the muscle fiber has to produce even more or it will shut down. Although there may be enough glucose to make ATP in the cell, if the oxygen in the bloodstream hasn't had time enough to arrive in sufficient quantities, a lesser form of fuel is produced for immediate energy needs called ADP. This type of energy is inefficient, and as a result, the muscle secrets more lactic acid, a toxic bi-product which is quite detrimental to any athletic performance. Occasionally, the energy demands of football, basketball, and intense track sports push you into this system. It's important in training to learn to minimize the amount of lactic acid secreted by the muscle while waiting for a sufficient oxygen supply to arrive from the heart to get back to ATP usage.

C. **The Aerobic System** (3 minutes and longer)

The properly developed aerobic system is characterized by efficient use of glucose and oxygen to produce ATP. Because it takes at least three to four minutes for sufficient amounts of oxygen to reach the muscle fiber, sports that demand a highly developed aerobic system are those that require long, sustained efforts.

These include sports such as long distance running, the longer tri-athalons, or long distance swimming or cycling. This energy system has only minimal application to the stop-and-go energy demands of football or basketball, but it is used as a base conditioning system for all sports. The major conditioning phase is the development of the cardiovascular system, accomplished by building the base through running or cross training thirty minutes and up to start with.

In order to develop each system most efficiently, you must be very specific about the type of endurance or overload stress that you place on the body. We will focus on an overall fitness model for our endurance-training program, and focus on all the energy systems.

How do we approach this when EVERYBODY is different? Why are we building this body? For general wellness, football, long distance running, or short, fast sprints?

Before we build a body we must know what we are building it for.

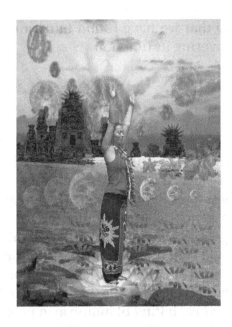

Chapter Two
The Organs of the Body

Glands

A gland is an organ or structure which either produces substances required by the body or eliminates waste substances from the body. Glands vary greatly in structure and size: some are mere pits or tiny depressions, some form sinuous, convoluted tubes, and others branch out like trees.

A sweat gland is an example of a small and simple gland. In contrast, the breast and the liver are larger, more complex glands. Some glands discharge their product directly into the blood or lymph. They are called endocrine or ductless glands. Others empty into a tube or duct which carries the product to the right place, as the pancreas does by discharging its secretion into the small intestine. Some glands have both functions, secreting one product into the blood and discharging another through a duct. The male sex glands (testicles) are in this class.

Of the glands that eliminate waste, the kidney is one of the best and most complex examples. Glands, especially ductless glands often work in teams, the action of one influencing that of the others. Some glands have the capacity to dominate the function of other glands. The most dominating of all glands is the pituitary gland (hypophysis), situated in the head at the base of the brain.

Over activity of a gland in most cases causes abnormal reactions in the body. An example is when the pituitary gland stimulates excessive growth, resulting in gigantism. Insufficient activity causes difficulties of another kind, as when the female sex glands slow down in their hormonal production, bringing on the various symptoms associated with menopause. Insufficient glandular activity can often be normalized by the administration either by mouth or by injection of the particular substances involved, as with thyroid extract.

Commonly used drugs, or now that we have found nutrition or other natural substances, often can assist the body in recovering its function.

Glands With Ducts

The Liver

This is a large gland or organ (the largest in the body) situated on the right side of the upper part of the abdomen. Its upper surface fits neatly under the diaphragm (the muscle which separates the abdomen and chest used in breathing). The under-surface of the liver fits over the right kidney. The liver has many important functions, hundreds in fact, so we will just cover a few major ones. It regulates the volume of the blood and stores iron and copper, which the body needs for use and function. The liver also produces substances, which keep the blood in a normal condition. The liver handles some poisonous substances that come from the intestines. It forms and secretes the bile, which aids in the absorption and digestion of fats. It regulates the quantity of each kind of amino acid present in the blood.

The amino acids are the building blocks of protein. The liver converts protein residue into urea, which is more suitable for elimination by the kidneys. It transforms glucose, a simple sugar that the body prefers to handle as fuel, into the more complex sugar, glycogen, which the liver stores for future use. When the body needs glucose, the liver breaks down the glycogen and releases it as glucose into the blood. The liver can be described as a kind of scavenger, since it helps (along with the spleen) in disposing of the residue from the breakdown of worn out red blood cells.

The liver stores a substance called heparin, which reduces the clotting (coagulating) tendency of the blood. It produces vitamin A from carotene. Extracts of liver are used to treat pernicious anemia, some forms of high blood pressure, a disease called sprue, etc.

The liver is a resilient organ but it is subject to many diseases, such as inflammation, tumors, overgrowth, hardening, withering, infection, etc. These are just a few of its numerous functions; it is a very important organ.

The Spleen

This organ is situated in the abdomen to the left and behind the stomach, directly under the diaphragm (the muscle separating the abdomen and chest). It is shaped somewhat like a kidney and is about 12 cm long.

The spleen destroys old red blood cells, liberating the pigment hemoglobin, which the liver converts to bilirubin, a constituent of bile. The spleen serves as a warehouse of active red blood cells, which it releases into the blood stream as needed during physical or emotional strain. The spleen is also capable of increasing and decreasing in size, thus it can vary the volume of blood in active circulation by withdrawing from or pouring into the blood stream. According to some researchers when fully expanded the spleen may hold as much as one third of the total volume of the blood in the body. This is why people in car accidents who rupture their spleens can bleed to death.

The Pancreas

A rather large, elongated gland situated in the left abdomen behind the stomach, and extending between the first part of the intestine and the spleen, the pancreas secretes a liquid containing four enzymes, which pass through a duct into the first part of the small intestine, the duodenum. It also produces the internal secretion insulin.

DIABETES

The following information is for educational purposes only and is meant to complement any medical treatment, not to prescribe or diagnose any condition. Please consult with your doctor before starting any medical or nutritional program.

With the invention of all our modern and refined processing for foods we have seen an increase in diabetes in our world. Some of the races that have diabetes in large numbers are the Hawaiians and the Native American Indians. Their bodies have a hard time adapting to the modern foods. More than any other disease, diabetes can be managed quite well with nutrition.

There are two types of diabetes: the first, diabetes insipidus, is more rare and has to do with a deficiency in the pituitary hormone called vasopressin. The other possibility is that the kidneys have an inability to respond properly to that hormone. People with this form of diabetes have several symptoms that make it stand out: they have tremendous thirst and they urinate large amounts regardless of how much they drink, and this shows us the weakness in the kidneys.

Diabetes Mellitus Type I is often called insulin-dependent diabetes It occurs at a young age and is sometimes called "Juvenile Diabetes." It is often caused by a viral attack on the system, but most experts are of the opinion that the body's immune system is weak when this occurs. With the destruction of the beta cells in the pancreas which manufactures the insulin, the body is unable to utilize glucose, the main food for the body. Consequently, the level of glucose is high in the blood since the body can't absorb it. This is often called "insulin resistance." The diabetic's blood becomes "too thick" or "sticky" and this causes blood clots or thromboses that damage blood vessels.

This can lead to the creation of excessive levels of free radicals (oxidants which break down the body faster) and makes the person more susceptible to the following problems: Diabetics have a larger risk of kidney disease, arteriosclerosis, blindness, heart disease or nerve diseases, as well as being more prone to infections. This is because of their body's resistance to insulin, which is the hormone that actually drives the glucose into the tissue and cells as a nutrient. When this does not happen the body becomes metabolically weak. The glucose molecules engage in an abnormal coupling with body proteins, a step called "glycosylation." Consequently, this disrupts the protein's ability to function biochemically and further weakens the immune system.

Some of the more common symptoms are abnormal thirst, again; irritability; weakness; fatigue; excessive urination; extreme loss of appetite or excessive hunger, and in the worst cases, vomiting and nausea. Some of these diabetics can have hyperglycemia type symptoms, which is too much glucose in their blood or at other times hypoglycemia when there is too low blood sugar. Both conditions can be serious. The worst of all these conditions is hypoglycemia, which can come from just missing a meal, or too much exertion or an insulin overdose. The symptoms could be dizziness, confusion, excessive sweating, and if not treated may lead to a coma. With hyperglycemia it could look the same as far as the symptoms, with not being able to keep down fluids as one of the danger signs. This means there is too much blood sugar in the system. It is more common during an illness and could also result in a coma. These two can be serious medical emergencies with life and death consequences.

A poor diet may be one of the biggest factors leading to diabetes. It often occurs with people who are overweight or who eat a diet high in refined sugar, highly processed foods, low in fiber, with too many complex carbohydrates and with too much meat, and who don't exercise.

The second category is Type II or non-insulin dependent diabetes, and more often occurs when people are older, and usually with people whose family may have a history of diabetes. This disorder is a little different in that the pancreas does produce insulin, but for some reason the insulin is not effective. Some of the common symptoms are poor vision; fatigue; frequent urination; skin infections, and slow healing of wounds as well as unusual thirst, drowsiness, and tingling or numbness in the feet. This disease is also linked to a poor diet. The National Institute of Health says that there are twenty to twenty-five million people with diabetes type problems, many have undetected Type II (some five million). Diabetes is the third leading cause of death in America. It can be detected with a simple urine test.

Nutrition

There is lots of controversy about nutrition but most experts agree that if there is excessive weight, a weight loss program is essential. Consult with a doctor who specializes in nutrition. As with other health challenges, each individual is different and I believe we need to treat the whole person. Many will recommend a high complex carbohydrate, low fat and high-fiber diet with lots of fresh vegetables, moderate fruits and green vegetable juices.

Excess fat cells create chemical messengers that block the body's ability to actually respond to the insulin. As the fat comes off the diabetic's own insulin works better and the blood sugar level can improve. Garlic and onion are always great for healing the body. Add some capsaicin, a natural derivative of hot peppers to spice it up and it is also very healthy.

Eat more steamed and raw vegetables, complex carbohydrates moderately, low fat foods (cut down on animal fats), and increase grains and whole foods. Avoid white flour, salt and white sugar as they elevate blood sugar levels. Eat more legumes, root vegetables, brown rice, and nut butters. Vegetable sources from protein are much better because high fiber helps reduce blood sugar urges. Eat proteins such as beans and tofu, salmon, and tuna two or three times a week. These fish have the Omega 3, great for the immune system. Eat lots of raw olive oil for your dressings or spread it on breads instead of butter; never use margarine.

Treat Cholesterol: High cholesterol increases the diabetic's risk for heart disease and stroke. Treat High Blood Pressure: Even modest blood pressure elevations greatly increase the risk of diabetes complications. Most diabetics should be compulsive about maintaining blood pressure control.

Plant fiber concentrates like psyllium (Metamucil, etc.) do more than just help with constipation problems. They can also help with absorption of sugar and starches. Some of these more common fibers have modest blood sugar lowering effects: glucomannan, guar gum, legume fiber, oat gum, pea fiber, apple pectin, and psyllium. Of course, the best way to get fiber is from increasing the fresh fruit and vegetables and legumes you eat so you get the fiber directly.

Avoid tobacco since it constricts your blood vessels and can be much more harmful to your condition. Eat more carbohydrates or reduce your insulin before exercise as it produces more insulin-like effect on the body. Exercise can cause low blood sugar (hypoglycemia) requiring a reduction in dose of insulin or diabetes pills. Diabetics with unrecognized heart disease are less likely than non-diabetics to feel chest pain (angina) as a warning sign that they are exercising too vigorously. (Consult with your doctor).

Most diabetics could cut down and eventually cut out their insulin or diabetes pills through a holistic program centered on nutrition. They could probably all benefit, reducing their risk of long term complications; however, you need to work with a medical doctor that uses nutrition in his or her practice.

Caution:

Many carbohydrates that people think of as being good for a diabetic can actually raise the glucose level of blood dramatically, e.g., whole wheat bread, many breakfast cereals, a baked potato, raisins, prunes or most dried fruit and carrot juice. Carrot juice is far too sweet. Better to juice a few little carrots and put in more greens such as kale, spinach, celery or wheat grass. Find a good green drink with many of the greens, which is also a great source of chlorophyll. Think: alkaline balance. Other carbohydrates such as pasta, pita bread, unleavened bread or bible bread, boiled potatoes, grapes, oranges, lemons or honeydew raise blood sugar only modestly.

Reduce the use of honey, molasses, etc. They do raise blood sugar, but most diabetics can tolerate them in small amounts, e.g., 1-2 tsp. a day if they are careful; however, it is better to try and do without. Replace those with fructose (fruit sugar) and lactose (milk sugar) as they do not raise blood sugar much and can be used in moderate amounts. A small percent of diabetics do not do well on a high carbohydrate diet, even one that is low in simple sugars and high in complex carbohydrates. Their blood sugar rises as do their triglycerides and cholesterol, so just increase the greens and legumes along with proteins.

Avoid fish oil capsules containing large amounts of para-amiobenzoic acid (PABA) as well as salt and white flour as they tend to raise blood sugar levels. Also, avoid taking large amounts of the amino acid cysteine because it can break down the bonds of the insulin hormone.

Mental Training

Mental calmness is critical for all health. Stress increases the adrenal glands' output of adrenaline and cortisone, two hormones which act to increase blood sugar. Relaxation training and stress management techniques help improve blood sugar control. Sometimes bio-feedback training could be very valuable -- see a professional.

Vitamins and Minerals

I recommend close medical supervision, for any treatment using vitamins or nutrition.

Chromium Picolinate, 400-600 mcg daily (Combination of chromium picolinate, vanadyl sulfate, and other vitamins and minerals that work together to regulate blood sugar levels), or
Diabetic Nutrition RX from Progressive Research Labs
Brewers yeast with added chromium can work too.
Biotin, 3-16 mg doses, but over 3 mg requires close medical supervision
Vitamin B-6, 50 mg. Take the B's together
Vitamin B1, 50-100 mg, Inositol, 50 mg daily
B-12 injection or lozenges- or sublingual for best results
Vitamin C, 1000-6000 mg
Calcium, 1000-1500 mg daily
Coenzyme Q10, 60-120 mg
L-Carnitine, L-Glutamine and Taurine, 500 mg of each (twice daily on empty stomach). Take with some Vitamin C for absorption, which mobilizes fat, reduces the craving for sugar, and aids in the release of insulin.
Manganese, 5-10 mg daily, do not take with calcium.
Magnesium, 600-700 mg
Quercetin, 100 mg 3 times per day
Vitamin E, 400-900 units
Zinc, 50-80 mg

In conclusion, regarding the emotions or how diabetics are living their lives from *The Wisdom of the Body:*

Diabetes people are living their life in an attitude of UNACCEPTABILITY of life at the most basic level (Sugars). They are never SATISFIED, never FULFILLED, and never CONTENT, they are always a work in progress.

Sources: Dr. James F. Balch, M.D., Phyllis A. Balch, C.N.C., and Dr. Richard Podell, M.D.

The last sentence taken from *Wisdom of the Body* by Roger Cotting, Dr. Diane Mistler (Misty), and Connie Smith, RN, about their work and teachings.

Parotid Glands

This pair of glands is responsible for secreting saliva. Each is located on the side of the head just below and in front of the ear. The parotid glands are the largest of the saliva glands; the other two are the sublingual and the submaxillary glands. They start digestion in the mouth.

Submaxillary Gland

A large saliva-producing gland situated below the back part of the lower jawbone, one on each side.

Sublingual Gland

One of two salivary glands situated on the floor of the mouth under the tongue, one on each side.

Lacrimal Glands

These glands produce tears. They are situated in the upper and outer part of the orbit (eye socket). The tear fluid runs from above and downward, thereby cleansing the surface of the eyeballs. The excess is drained either through the nasolacrimal duct into the nose or through the "tear ducts" at the inner angle of the eyelids.

Mammary Glands

The breast, or milk-secreting organs of female. The human breast consists of about fifteen to twenty-five secreting units embedded in a cushion of fat supported by a network of connective tissue. Each unit, which looks somewhat like a bunch of grapes, begins at the periphery of the breast (as from the rim of a wheel) and extends like a spoke toward the nipple (the hub). As each unit or lobe converges towards the nipple, the amount of glandular or secreting tissue diminishes (like the wedge of a pie). These fine milk-carrying ducts combine to form a stalk-like outlet (lactiferous duct) in the nipple. There are as many lactiferous ducts as there are lobes or units in the breast. Each opens through a small pore in the nipple. The milk can really pour out of the nipple.

Sebaceous Glands

Glands which produce sebum, a fatty, lubricating material. These glands are located mainly in the skin and are especially abundant around the lower and outer part of the nose.

Suderiferus Glands

These are the glands which produce or convey sweat (the sweat glands).

The Reproductive Glands

The organs and structures concerned with reproduction. In the male these consist of the penis, testicles, prostate, seminal vesicles, Cowper's glands and various ducts. In the female the system consists of the vagina, uterus, uterine tubes and ovaries.

Ductless Glands

The Thyroid

A large endocrine or ductless organ situated in front of and on both sides of the windpipe (trachea), or throat. It consists essentially of two lobes, one on either side and a connecting portion below called the isthmus. The main product of the gland is called thyroxin, which regulates the body's growth. Absence of the gland at birth causes a condition known as cretinism. Deficiency of its activity causes myxedema.

Parathyroids

Small glands (usually four in number) situated near the thyroid gland. They secrete a hormone that regulates the calcium content of the blood.

Intestinal Glands

Small glands situated in the lining membrane of the intestine, the digestive tube, which extends from the outlet of the stomach to the outlet of the body at the anus. The first part is the small intestine. Partially digested food empties from the stomach into the small intestine where the digestive process is completed. By peristalsis (rhythmical muscular contractions) the food matter is moved through the intestinal tract and nourishment is absorbed through the wall of the small intestine into the lymph and blood. By the time the matter reaches the large intestine, it is mostly waste.

The Small Intestine

It starts at the stomach and runs in irregular coils for more than 20 feet where it empties into the large intestine in the right, lower part of the abdomen. The small intestine is arbitrarily divided into three parts, starting at the stomach: the duodenum, the jejunum, and the ileum.

The Large Intestine

The large intestine is about five feet long and begins in the right, lower part of the abdomen (where the appendix is) runs up and then across to the left side, and finally down, ending at the anus. Its form resembles a question mark. The large intestine is also arbitrarily divided into three parts, starting at the end of the small intestine: the cecum, the colon, and the rectum. The anus is the outlet of the rectum. The large intestine concentrates the residue, extracts most of the water, and then ejects it as feces.

The Lungs

These are the breathing organs in which the blood receives oxygen and releases carbon dioxide. There are two lungs, a right and a left, situated in the thorax or chest. The interior of the chest may be envisioned as the upper half of an upright barrel, separated from the lower half by a horizontal sheet of rubber (representing the diaphragm). The shape of each lung is more or less like that of a bullet with its rounded or pointed end up. However, the lung is not a round structure. In cross-section, near the middle it is rather hemispherical or semi-lunar, like a lug split lengthwise. The rounded side of each lung fits the inner contour of the sides of the chest. The flattened sides of the lungs, which are really somewhat concave or hollowed, face each other at the midline of the chest. The space between the two hollowed surfaces of the lungs is known as the mediastinum, which is a space of considerable size.

The mediastinum extends from the breastbone in the front to the spine in the back. It extends from the diaphragm below to the ceiling of the interior of the chest below the clavicle. The diaphragm is the muscular sheet that separates the chest from the abdomen. The mediastinum contains the heart and its great blood vessels, the aorta and the vena cava. It also contains the esophagus (the tube which conveys swallowed food from the mouth to the stomach), the trachea (or windpipe) which brings in the air to the lungs, and other smaller structures.

The left lung, which is smaller than the right, is divided into two lobes, the superior lobe and the inferior lobe by a fissure or groove. The right and larger lung is divided into three lobes, the superior lobe, middle lobe and inferior lobe. Smaller subdivisions are based on the branching of the bronchial tubes within the lung tissue.

A thin membrane called the visceral pleura covers the entire outer surface of the lungs. At the root of the lung, this membrane turns back and lines the internal surface of the corresponding side of the chest, forming the parietal pleura. This configuration may be replicated by pushing the fist into the side of a slightly inflated balloon. The rubber layer that surrounds the fist can represent the visceral pleura. The second layer (that lines the inner surface of the chest) is the parietal pleura. In the case of the balloon there is an air-filled space between the two layers of rubber.

In the chest, the two layers of membrane, the visceral pleura and the parietal pleura, are in close contact, separated only by a thin layer of skin and lubricating fluid. Only when the chest wall is pierced, surgically or accidentally and the lung collapses does the space between the two layers of pleura become of considerable size.

These capillaries are in close contact with the finest divisions of the bronchial tubes, the air carrying system. The finest subdivisions of the air carrying system are called pulmonary (i.e. lung) alveoli. These are tiny sacs on the ends and sides of the bronchial tube branches. They may be envisioned as a bunch of seedless grapes wherein the stalk and its branches represent the finest subdivisions of the bronchial tubes. In other words, one may imagine that the stalk, its branches, and the grapes are hollow and contain air; this would represent a unit of lung tissue. Coursing around the thin skins of the grapes are the capillaries of the blood vessels. It is here where the vital transfer of oxygen and carbon dioxide occurs in this delicate link between the capillaries (the finest branches of the blood vessels) and the "grapes" (the pulmonary alveoli) where breathing takes place.

The oxygen leaves the "grapes" and enters the capillaries. The carbon dioxide leaves the capillaries and enters the "grapes" or pulmonary alveoli. The blood is now clean and oxygenated; the foul air in the lung is exhaled out through the mouth.

The purpose of respiration is to bring the blood and the air close together, separated by only a thin barrier of tissue, thus allowing the carbon dioxide of the "used" blood to be expelled and allowing fresh oxygen to enter the blood and refresh it. The exchange takes place in the lung tissue where the finest branches of the blood vessels are separated from the finest subdivisions of the bronchial tubes by a layer of cells, which permit the passage of carbon dioxide and oxygen, the breath of life.

ASTHMA

First of all, I want to make it clear that this information is not to diagnose nor to prescribe and it should not take the place of the advice of your doctor. This is intended to complement conventional medicine, not to replace it. Consult with your doctor before starting any kind of nutritional or physical program.

Asthma is considered a spasm or inflammation of the bronchial tubes that lead to the lungs. This can be due to irritation caused by allergies to food or airborne pollution, or a sensitivity that is out of what we call the "norm." This sensitivity could be to all the above or it can be emotional. Some researchers think it could be an inherited or genetic weakness. I have not seen enough research for this to be substantiated, so I leave that up to the experts. I do know, however, it can happen at any age yet it is more common during childhood and some kids just outgrow it. About 6 to 7% of the population has asthma, and it seems to be more common among males.

There is a lot of controversy about asthma. The main problem is not taking a breath in but in releasing the breath out. If we look at this from a psychological standpoint it has to do with letting go of certain attitudes, or holding on to certain emotions. We know that certain stress increases an asthmatic's condition or can even bring about an attack. What this is telling many of us is that asthma can be very much tied in with our minds and emotions. I know this from some of the latest research I have read and from having an asthmatic son and stepson. I was able to put many medical and natural remedies to work with my own family.

There is much to learn about asthma and whether or not nutritional approaches can really help this condition. In my experience, asthma can be as different as the patient that has it, and every case needs to be looked at separately. I feel very strongly about this approach with all symptoms or diseases. We need to treat the whole person and not lump everyone into the same category of asthmatics, for example.

We do know that many asthmatics seem to have airborne allergies and/or sensitivity to foods. Often times the traditional allergy tests like skin or blood tests can confirm certain serious allergies. However, it's some of the not so commonly recognized food allergies that may be the problem. By just eliminating commonly known allergens such as dairy products, wheat, peanuts, excessive sugar, and according to other nutritional doctors, certain shellfish, shrimp and sulfates, which seem to irritate the mucous lining, I know most will improve.

Eliminating dairy products would be beneficial if the person gets excessive mucus when ingesting them. Wheat is a common allergen for most people because the gluten is very hard to digest. There are very good alternative sources for calcium such as many green leafy vegetables, cabbage, and cauliflower, as well as sunflower seeds and almonds. You can purchase soy milk, almond milk or rice milk; these alternative products are less mucus forming. Once again, every individual is different. Care must be used if certain foods are eliminated and then introduced again because there may be a harsher reaction to them the second time around.

Here in Hawaii, we have another problem -- molds, mildew and airborne allergens such as pollen and certain dusts. Some asthmatics are allergic to ordinary house dust. If your child has sensitivities to these pollutants there are air purifiers, ionizing machines, etc. that can be of benefit in the home. When I had my son tested for allergies there were even couch dust allergies that affected him. You may want to get dehumidifiers for their bedroom. All of these things can help.

If we look at the work by Dr. Robert Young about having the body be more alkaline, we can see that many of the problems occur with food choices. The body can do quite well on a diet low in protein and high in greens, vegetables, and a little carbohydrate. I find the key is to get some expert advice if you are not a nutritionist, and none of this information is meant to replace seeing your doctor for asthma. Hopefully, it will complement and educate you to alternative approaches. Care should be taken in any change of diet and with the use of medicines or even herbs.

Many allergies to dairy products, bread or yeast, and even to eggs or corn are hard to test for in the laboratory. Many times the reaction is very subtle and not so obvious. Changing one's diet will take time before seeing any results. You will not see dramatic results on a long term condition in a few short months. Once again, you should think of consulting a nutritional doctor for the best way to approach this condition.

Nutritional Approach

Foods to Eliminate or Cut Down On

Look for specific asthma triggers that produce, for example, excess mucus. If after eating a pizza, the kid gets a runny nose and starts to cough for the next two days, this may tell you something. This is an obvious one but many times we don't pay close attention and there are many more subtle triggers. Foods that create a lot of gas can cause pressure on the diaphragm and sometimes trigger an asthma attack as well, so watch for that.

Eliminate or greatly reduce potential allergens such as the dairy products and replace with almond milk or soy products. Buy unyeasted breads, eliminate wheat, barley and rye gluten products, and cut out peanuts. Reduce or eliminate sodas and sweets, even reduce fruit that is too concentrated with natural sugars such as dried fruit. Juices should always be watered down for kids, anyway. Reduce salt intake and cut out artificial sweeteners, and check your labels for additives and other unnatural colors, etc. More natural foods are better for everyone, not just asthmatics. A low salt diet may reduce bronchial sensitivity and improve asthma status as well. Remember, work with the child on all levels because emotional distress is also an important asthma trigger that is often overlooked.

For Adults

The same recommendations apply as far as eliminating the foods above. Alcohol varies in its effect on individual asthmatics; it can help some (I think it calms them) or make it worse. Often it conflicts with digestion. Wine may make the condition worse because of the many sulfates used in making it.

Caffeine can have a modest, acute anti-asthma relief, probably because of its chemical similarity to the asthma medicine, Theophylline. However, I wouldn't recommend using coffee. It should be reduced because of its high acidity. Teas could be used. I'm not fanatical about anything, but coffee on an empty stomach does not help the body, and if you are asthmatic you already have an overly sensitive body.

Foods

As I said earlier, eat lots of greens; they are great for the body. The key is to try and eliminate acid foods like meats, bread, sweets, and dairy products. Broccoli is one of the best vegetables because it is 65% protein. Eat more avocados; they are not fattening and they have the good fats (see nutrition article). Now there are green drinks on the market with many grasses that are very high in chlorophyll. Work with a specialist to get your body back to an alkaline balance. It is the strongest protection for the immune system. Eat more onions and garlic with your food. Reduce meat protein and increase protein such as tofu or fish, tuna and salmon being among the best because they are high in Omega 3 as well as fish oil, which has a powerful anti-inflammatory effect and a benefit found in treating rheumatoid arthritis. It may be helpful for asthma as well. These stimulate and heal the immune system. Use sea kelp for minerals and seasoning.

Bee pollen has proved to be helpful if eaten from local sources. If the allergies are airborne, bee pollen can strengthen the immune system and the body will start to resist the pollens it's allergic to. Be sure to start with a few granules at a time and work up to two or three teaspoons daily. It's great in smoothies. Discontinue if rashes or wheezing occur using those small amounts.

Herbs

(Caution! All herbs are like medicine and should not be taken for long term use unless you are consulting with your doctor.)

The best herbs or natural foods are garlic and onions but gingko biloba known best for its benefit on the mind or its "anti-senility" effects may help. During an attack, I used a lobelia, goldenseal and bee propolis tincture that worked great for the kids, not for long term use, though. Other herbs that are beneficial are mullein oil in tea or juice, slippery elm tea or tablets, horsetail, juniper berries, licorice root and Pau d'arco tea.

Ma huang, a Chinese herb (ephedra sinica), can be used as a tea twice daily but it's not recommended for extended use. This plant is a source of the asthma medicine, ephedrine, a close cousin of Theophylline, a widely used asthma medicine. Most doctors recommend the use of the prescription medicines Theophylline or ephedrine since the potency of the tea is not consistent and can have serious side effects like nervousness and irregular heart beat.

Tylophora asthmatica in tea twice daily can be taken but it is not recommended for long term use, either. This Indian herb has been used to treat asthma in the Ayurvedic tradition for thousands of years.

Quercitin, 500 mg 3 times daily, is an important bioflavonoid, and is biochemically similar to the anti-asthma drug Intalcromolyn. In some experiments quercitin has been shown to prevent mast cells from releasing histamines, a chemical that aggravates allergic reactions.

Vitamins (Recommended doses are for adults or large teenagers)

Very helpful, for most of us as well are most anti-oxidant vitamins. Vitamin A, 10,000 -20,000 IU daily; 10,000 -20,000 IU's daily of natural beta carotene. Vitamin C, 1500-3000 mg daily. Always take Vitamin C with bioflavinoids, one of the lungs most important anti-oxidant defenses. High doses can be given to asthmatics before an acute exposure to irritants or allergens. Vitamin B complex, 500-1000 mg daily with extra Vitamin B-6, 50-200 mg daily; Niacin (vitamin B-3) or niacinamide; Bromelain (Wobenzime from Maryln Nutriceudicals), 1000 -3000 mg daily. Bromelain is a pineapple enzyme. I'm a great believer in this nutrient for many things. It is a natural anti-inflammatory nutrient, reducing inflammation not only in the joints but it also works on the lungs. Also, pycnogenol or grape seed extract is both anti-inflammatory and an anti-oxidant. Magnesium, 300-600 mg (magnesium helps an acute asthma attack when given intravenously.) Most nutrition oriented physicians believe oral magnesium can help chronic asthma as well. Vitamin D, 500 IU daily. N-Acetyl Cysteine, 500-1000 mg. This nutrient is converted in the body to glutathione. It has definite mucous thinning and anti-oxidant effects.

Vitamin B-12, orally 1,000 mcg twice a day or for some acute conditions, an injection of Vitamin B-12, 1000 mcg weekly may be helpful (see your physician)

Amino acids l-cysteine, 500 mg twice a day on an empty stomach taken with the B vitamins and Vitamin C. Along with that, also take l-methionine, 500 mg twice a day.

Recommendation

Consult an allergist and get a food test (cytotoxic) and a skin test (intracutaneous titration). Some doctors even do the sublingual provocation and pulse tests to determine your food allergies or other airborne allergies. Always keep in mind that the interpretation of these tests is highly subjective often depending on the doctor that you are working with. Find one that also works with nutrition.

Often times it's more accurate to eliminate suspected foods and to keep a food diary to identify trigger foods. Watch your child's food or your own carefully. Consider eliminating the other potentially common allergen foods but only in a well-supervised approach, and be prepared to treat an acute asthma reaction when reintroducing suspected foods.

A good example of an elimination diet could be eating many of the greens in salads, brown rice, sweet potatoes, squash, or for us in Hawaii, poi, which is made from taro, a great food and hypo-allergenic to most people. Then, of course, many steamed vegetables can be eaten such as beets and their greens, asparagus, chard, squash, carrots, artichokes, string beans and spinach. Very small amounts of cooked fruits such as peaches, apricots, papaya, plums and prunes. No citrus fruits. Cooking fruits alters the protein in them making them less likely to be allergens. Then after a cleansing diet, re-introduce some of these foods, one at a time on an empty stomach, to see the results.

Take an insurance formula multi-vitamin/mineral. The best ones are liquid and they should be specific for age and weight. Listed above are doses meant for an adult or a large teenager.

Consider also a six-week trial of 1000 mcg vitamin B-12 injections for the children.

There is a good source for many of these nutrients called "Urban Air Defense" from Source Naturals, a great company.

I hope this information has been helpful to you but it is not meant to replace your doctor. Always be sure to check with your physician before undergoing any severe change in your diet or in your children's diet.

Sources:
Richard Podell, M.D., Andrew Weil, M.D., John McDougall, M.D., James F. Balch, M.D., and Phyllis Balch, C.N.C.

The Heart

Used blood is depleted of oxygen and impregnated with the waste product carbon dioxide and other byproducts. This blood may be regarded as "sewage," flowing through the veins inward to the sewage processing plant, the lungs, via the heart. All returning blood is poured into the right side of the heart, which consists of the upper auricle (or atrium) and the lower ventricle. The right ventricle is the muscular chamber whose contractions send the used carbon dioxide-rich blood into the lung by way of the pulmonary arteries. Within the lung these large blood vessels divide and subdivide until they become slender capillaries, which have thin and permeable walls.

The blood, which has now been refreshed, continues the course in the blood vessels of the lung. Now these vessels unite here and there to form larger vessels instead of dividing and becoming thinner as they did before taking on the oxygen. The blood within these vessels is now fresh blood. The vessels are called veins rather than arteries (which carry fresh blood elsewhere in the body) because they carry blood to the heart. The refreshed blood is finally poured into the left side of the heart by way of the pulmonary veins. The left side of the heart, like the right, consists of an upper atrium (or auricle) and a lower ventricle. The muscular contractions of the left ventricle are produced by the largest of the heart muscles, propelling the oxygen-fresh blood through the aorta and its branches to all parts of the body. The cycle continues as this blood releases its oxygen to the tissues, taking on carbon dioxide, and returning to the right side of the heart and then to the lungs again.

This is the endless cycle by which the blood is repeatedly "polluted" in the body tissues and "cleansed" in the lungs. This is the role played by the blood and the circulatory system, the heart and blood vessels. The heart is the most amazing organ, and we are just starting to fully understand its many functions.

The Kidneys

The kidneys are two complex organs which form urine from toxic material removed from the blood. They are situated on each side of the spine in the back part of the abdomen. Each kidney is about 11 cm long, 6 cm wide and 2.5 cm thick.

The kidneys form the urine from the liquid portion of the blood and from the waste material dissolved in it. To accomplish this, the blood is circulated through the kidneys in a continuous stream. The work of the kidney is done by a large number (perhaps a million) of "filtering" units called nephrons. Each unit pours its product into a funnel-shaped part of the kidney called the pelvis. From the pelvis the urine is carried to the bladder by a tube called the urethra.

Each filtering unit (nephron) is composed of a tuft (glomerulus) of very thin blood capillaries brought in contact with a urine collecting tube or tubule. There is no opening between the capillaries and the collecting tubule, otherwise whole blood would pass. There is merely a close contact between the walls of the collecting tubule and those of the capillaries, similar to the alveoli in the lungs. The fluid with the waste matter in it passes from the blood through the capillary walls and into the collecting tubule by passing through its wall.

To visualize how they actually touch, imagine a pear-shaped, rubber ear syringe compressed between the two fingers and the thumb. The invaginated bulb of the syringe is very much like the closed end of the collecting tubule, which is expanded and also invaginated. The tuft of capillaries lies snugly sheltered in this hollow as a small ball in the cupped palm and fingers of the hand. The tuft of capillaries and the expanded end of the collecting tubule in the hollow in which it lies is called the Malpighian corpuscle.

Inflammation of the kidney or deterioration of the substance of its delicate structure is called nephritis. Inflammation of the pelvis of the kidney is called pyelitis. Our kidneys work very hard to excrete toxins from the body.

The Thymus

A mass of tissue, possibly a gland of internal secretion (i.e., endocrine gland) situated in the upper part of the chest cavity along the windpipe (trachea). It's larger in the early years of childhood and decreases in size after puberty. The function of the thymus is not clearly understood, but we know it has a lot to do with the immune system.

The Adrenal Glands

The adrenal glands are also called suprarenal glands. They are endocrine (internal secretion) glands situated above the kidneys, one on each side. Each gland is composed of an internal portion called the medulla, covered by the external cortex. These portions may be visualized as the flesh and the rind of a fruit. The medulla produces epinephrine, a substance that raises blood pressure. The outer cortex produces the adrenal cortical hormones.

The Pituitary Gland (or Hypophysis)

The hypophysis is without a doubt the most important gland in the body. It is a small, oval ductless (endocrine) gland situated at the base of the brain, consisting of two lobes, an anterior and a posterior. The anterior (front) lobe secretes several important hormones that regulate the function of other important glands such as the thyroid, the adrenals, the testes, the ovaries, etc. Its role is therefore crucial in the growth, maturation, and reproductive activity of an individual. A stalk to another part of the brain called the hypothalamus attaches the pituitary gland. Improper function of the posterior lobe may result in a condition called diabetes insipidus (not to be confused with the more common form of diabetes.)

The Skin

The skin is the largest organ in the body. It is our outermost covering and consequently is at high risk of being damaged, injured, cut, and infected. It literally keeps us together, holding all the muscles and organs inside. It also helps to keep us warm and cool. It's amazing how well the skin stands up to a constant attack of germs, dirt, pollution, scrapes, bangs, friction, sun, wind, heat, and cold. There are reasons why your skin lasts so long and can stay in fairly good shape. Skin cells are constantly replaced; the old ones slough off as new cells are produced. You grow a new surface layer of skin every 28 days or so. If you cut yourself, the skin will grow up to seven times faster to repair itself. (Our white cells not only fight infection but also help build and repair tissue.)

The skin is specially adapted in many ways to resist infection. It maintains a dry outer surface that prevents the accumulation of germs and bacteria, unlike wetness and warmth, which promote their growth. Many problems with skin or bacterial infection can be avoided with sun and saltwater just by jumping in the ocean. The skin can adapt to many environments. In cold climates we perspire less and in warmer climates we sweat more to cool the body. It also can defend itself from intense use. If the skin is frequently and vigorously rubbed, as in manual labor or many sports, it will protect itself by forming the thick covering we know as a callus.

Fibromyalgia or Myofascial Pain Syndrome

First of all, I want to make it clear that this information is not to diagnose nor to prescribe and it should not take the place of the advice of your doctor. This is intended to complement conventional medicine, not to replace it. Consult with your doctor before starting any kind of nutritional or physical program, especially if you have been diagnosed with fibromyalgia.

What is fibromyalgia? There has been much confusion about this condition in part because it has been given many names. It used to be called fibrositis, or myofascial pain, myofascial pain syndrome, psychogenic rheumatism, fibromyositis, myofasciitis, tensionmyalgia, or psychological muscle disorder. It has frequently been confused with CMFS, chronic muscular fatigue syndrome.

Many people think it's a very new disease but it has been recognized for some 100 years or longer. Only recently have we used the terms fibromyalgia or myofascial pain syndrome as the most acceptable definitions. Fibromyalgia syndrome is the most common term due to the many associated symptoms found with this disorder.

Chronic muscular pain is just one facet of this syndrome; it runs much deeper than just sore and aching muscles or joints. Just living with gravity and our modern day stress can cause much of the soreness and muscle tension that most people experience. However, when we have the condition of fibromyalgia, or myofascial pain syndrome, all of the stress and tension is intensified ten-fold.

The chronic pain can be regional, myofascial pain syndrome (in the connective tissue or muscles) or widespread fibromyalgia with overall aches and pains accompanied by neurological and other problems. The condition can be very severe and has many faces. There is a lot of controversy surrounding fibromyalgia, mainly because it is so hard to diagnose, with each person having different symptoms and pains. My theory is that the weak link in any body will determine the type of symptoms the patient shows as well as the severity of the condition. Thus it is critical to understand the whole person, the individual and their lifestyle to determine how to approach their wellness and provide the best treatment. Our approach is to treat each individual holistically and work with the whole person and not just the symptom.

What happens with fibromyalgia and myofascial pain syndrome?

Since mostly women suffer from fibromyalgia, most experts think it is connected to the hormone estrogen. It could be an estrogen insufficiency or certain hormonal changes that affect the muscle pain. It's usually found in women over thirty.

It's interesting that the disease of fibromyalgia is mostly a female disease and I suspect someday we may find an underlying hormonal relationship. I have never heard of males with this condition in my thirty years of experience. I have known only a few women that actually were diagnosed with this condition. It probably is not just about a high or low level of hormones, but how the nervous system and muscle tissue is affected by these hormonal imbalances. It could be heredity, but there is not sufficient research in this area yet.

There was a study at the Ohio State University in 1989 by Pellegrino. He suggested that fibromyalgia is an inherited problem. In other words, half the children of fibromyalgia sufferers could potentially develop the disease. In the few cases I have seen, I didn't find that to be true as compared to scoliosis of which I saw many more cases. I think scoliosis was more common with women and most patients' mothers had it as well.

Some of the Common Symptoms of FMS

Intense Pain The pain of fibromyalgia is different in every individual and has no limits; sometimes it's a dull pain and other times sharp. It can be numbness on the surface of the skin or deep, muscular aching that is dull, shooting, burning, throbbing or stabbing, sharp pain. Most often, the pain and stiffness are worse in the morning, and it's not unusual to hurt in the muscle groups that are used more often: upper neck, shoulders, low back, hips, and legs. In fact, often every joint may hurt. Here again it varies with the person. Their activities or jobs, as well as their mechanical postures, can dictate where they will suffer most.

Chronic Fatigue This symptom can be mild in some patients and totally incapacitating for others. The fatigue has been described as "feeling unmotivated" or "having mental fatigue." Some patients told me if they could get the strength to get out of bed then they could deal with the rest of the day. But just getting out of bed is a challenge (see sleep disorders). Often they feel totally drained of energy. Some patients feel like their arms and legs are heavy, movement takes great effort, and often they have difficulty concentrating because the mind is fatigued as well as the body.

Chronic Headaches Recurrent migraine or tension type headaches are seen in about 50-60% of fibromyalgia patients and can pose a major problem. Just dealing with the daily activities of life can be a struggle for these patients.

Sleep Disorders Most fibromyalgia patients have a sleep disorder called the alpha-EEG anomaly. This means that they don't get to the deeper levels of sleep and they are constantly interrupted by awakening brain activity. Thus, when they wake up they feel that they didn't get any rest and the body did not get a chance to recover. This condition creates added stress, which keeps them in the vicious cycle. One of my patients said she felt like she'd been run over by a truck when she got up every morning; everything hurt and many days she just didn't want to get out of bed.

Temperomandibular Joint Dysfunction Syndrome (TMJ) This syndrome is connected with the headaches or face pain in 25-30% of FMS patients. Research indicates that as many as 90% of fibromyalgia patients may have jaw and facial tenderness that could produce the same symptoms of TMJ. So we assume that most of the problems associated with this condition related to the muscles and ligaments holding the jaw together.

Irritable Bowel Syndrome (IBS) It's common for many of these women to have bowel problems, constipation or diarrhea. Frequent abdominal or chest pain is also not uncommon. These symptoms are found in 60% to 70% of fibromyalgia patients, according to the research, in addition to PMS and painful menstrual periods (dysmenorrhea).

Some patients with chronic fatigue syndrome (CFS) have the alpha-EEG sleep pattern disorder, and some fibromyalgia-diagnosed patients have been found to have other sleep disorders as well. Most common is Myoclonus or PLMS (nighttime jerking of the arms and legs), restless leg syndrome, and bruxism (teeth grinding). The sleep pattern for clinically depressed patients is distinctly different from that found in patients with FMS or CFS.

Other common symptoms include muscle numbness and or tingling sensations; muscle twitching; swollen extremities, dry skin or skin sensitivity, dry eyes and mouth; dizziness and impaired coordination. Often patients experience sensitivity to weather or wind, rain, and changes in temperature. Hormonal fluctuations (premenstrual and menopausal states), depression, anxiety and overexertion can all contribute to symptom flare-ups.

There are four main components that we see in most of these patients. Understanding them is important to optimize healing in a holistic approach.

Recurring injury in the form of micro-trauma and biomechanical imbalances perpetuate muscle strain. This means that if your body is out of alignment, along with having this condition, you are setting up micro-injuries by stressing the muscle and connective tissue constantly. This pain/stress cycle can create over use syndrome, which will tax the body's ability to deal with pain.

1. Pain sensitivity is turned way up. The central nervous system changes induced by constant muscle strains that "turn up" the sensitivity to pain create heightened stress, chemically as well as neurologically. This condition is often called Allodynia. This usually makes normal people react abnormally to low levels of painful stimuli that would previously not have caused much stress. The body can normally handle this, even though many people will have sore and tense muscles. These changes are physical as well as physiological. The body has to release more histamines, endorphins, and other anti-inflammatory chemicals to just keep

the balance. Eventually the body gives up because it cannot keep up with the unusual demand and intensity.

2. Nerve propreoceptive tissue increases in size. According to recent research, the nerve propreoceptive cells that carry pain messages from the muscles to the spine, and eventually to the brain, actually increase in size as chronic pain persists. If not an actual increase in size, the irritation caused to the nerves creates this hyper-sensitivity not only on the skin and muscles but all the way into the joints and organs as well. Serotonin (a soothing chemical in the body) in the central nervous system falls, and this can increased Substance P, which is an inflammatory neurochemical and causes more pain when it's released. Thus a physiological (chemical) change as well starts to happen in the body. Some of the brain imaging tests with highly sophisticated equipment such as fluoroscopes show pain pathways "lighting up" at just moderate levels of pressure on skin and muscle that would not normally show before the allodynia process had set in. This means that mild pressure on a normal subject is much more intense on a person with this condition. We advocate very gentle massage for soothing relief, but more importantly for balancing the body mechanics to reduce the stress and reach the deeper cause of muscle irritability.

3. There is increased vulnerability to other disorders. Naturally, a body that is under severe stress and constantly fighting with pain is more susceptible as the immune system weakens from over exertion. Neuro-chemical, metabolic, and hormonal overload causes the increased vulnerability to other diseases and conditions, especially any biochemical abnormalities that could overlap with the myofascial pain and fibromyalgia. This is where diagnosis can become difficult. As the body weakens from the overload, the weakest link is the first to manifest a problem. Just as a viral flu will hit people in different places - some get the throat soreness, some cough in the lungs, and others get stomach disorder -- they all arise from the same virus.

4. The chronic pain undermines health. This constant pain puts the body on full alert, and over a prolonged period of time it can cause problems with the immune system as well. Due to the complications of chronic pain and how it undermines both physical and mental health in most people, we need to assist our patients at the frontline of wellness. Continued stress could out-picture with lost appetite or increased eating disorders; disrupted sleep; weakened immune resistance; inadequate exercise; increased craving for sugar; discouragement and depression. Each can lead to the body not functioning at its optimum level.

Holistic Treatment

The holistic approach seeks to approach the problem on all levels-- mental, nutritional, and physical. Each aspect of these problems needs a specific modality or therapy. We recommend the use of conventional medicine with nutritional, herbal, biochemical nutrients, bio-mechanical body therapy, and mind-body methods designed to enhance the body's own natural healing systems.

Nutritional and Herbal Treatments

We know that the best way to approach a vague disease is to use conventional holistic practices such as good nutrition, lower fat intake (especially the saturated fats), less sugar and fewer junk foods. Increase water intake for flushing the system and increase intake of anti-oxidants Vitamins C, E, beta carotene, and a good multi-vitamin, with increased doses of cell salts and selenium. Some medical experts say phosphatigylserine, which is a lipid (fat processor) and gingko biloba can also help ease the condition. Also, adding fish oil capsules.

From a natural perspective, GABA itself is available from the health food stores over the counter. Again, I just want to caution anyone self-medicating, even with natural substances.

Magnesium-calcium and selenium supplements also may help by acting on some of the same neural and muscle receptor sites that GABA influences.

About 80% of our chronic pain patients are deficient in magnesium. That's because physical pain (and also mental anguish) cause the muscles to overwork and the muscles use up much more magnesium than normal. This is a reason why many athletes need extra magnesium as well.

Ironically, the muscles really need that magnesium to function and not having enough of it increases muscle spasm and pain, as well as the general vulnerability to stressful stimuli such as loud noises, chemicals, and emotional distress. So this hyper-sensitivity puts people in that kind of vicious cycle.

Many of these patients have hypoglycemia or blood sugar control problems as well. This is normally due to the stress of their illness on the glucose/insulin system. Excess stress causes the body to be on high alert. Consequently, the dietary guidelines described above could be very helpful in conjunction with a few quick and helpful nutritional tricks. A small supplementation of olive oil, chromium, or glutamine can usually reverse this common complication. Once again, be sure to not just approach the symptom but to work with the whole person.

Of course we know that sleep is crucial for natural healing. The latest studies show that fibromyalgia pain can be produced in just a single night. When the sleeping person is just jostled at a specific sector of the EEG dream cycle, even if they continue to sleep without being awakened, they will not get the deep rest they need for healing.

Natural remedies to help sleep are valerian root, 5-hydroxy tryptophan, passion flower, GABA, and melatonin. Relaxation or meditation training and other natural approaches can do much to restore good sleep. This is a bit more complicated than it sounds; we advise that you consult with a professional. Of course, some medicines can also help with sleep as long as care is taken to not create a habit or dependence on these drugs. Reducing alcohol as well as reducing caffeine and sugar will help the body sleep better.

Conventional Medicines

The most interesting recent research is that the kinds of medicine that work best for fibromyalgia and myofascial pain are not the traditional narcotic pain suppressors such as vicodine, codeine, or the highly potent, non-steroidal, anti-inflammatory medicines such as Celebrex or muscle relaxers such as Flexeril.

The best medicines acrording to Dr. Podell to use instead are those that act on our nervous system and neurochemistry to reduce and reverse allodynia, the body's abnormal increased sensitivity to that pain.

None of these new medicines is a cure by itself since they don't always get to the original cause, which we really don't understand. As we mentioned before, every individual is different and there is no magic pill that will work for everyone. Many of the drugs do have some potential side effects. However, with a clear approach to strengthening the patient by using the holistic approach, the body can heal much more than we give it credit. The key is patience by both patient and doctor and especially keeping an open mind and looking at all the healing choices available. We can almost always find one, two or three safe tools as well as effective drugs or nutrients that can help reduce the pain and the vulnerability to further problems, and hopefully without undue side effects or increased stress. If we start early enough, many things help. The problem is that most people don't seek medical help until they have had it for years.

The most surprising news is that many of the best new medicines are actually old standbys that have been used for many years for other conditions. Because of the complexity of fibromyalgia, we are just re-discovering the beneficial effects for helping the neuro-chemistry. Some of the common medicines used are Baclofen, Elavil, Flexeril, Gabatril, Klonopin, Neurontin, Paxil, Sinequan, Serzone, Xanax, and Zofran.

Baclofen is commonly used for muscle relaxation with people that have multiple sclerosis. Baclofen enhances the GABA neuro-transmitters that help reduce the central nervous system pain and also relax the muscles.

Neurontin and Gabatril are two more GABA enhancers that were first used to treat patients with epileptic seizures. These can also help chronic nervous disorders and muscle pain.

Zaniflex is another muscle relaxant (first used for multiple sclerosis) that can reduce the body's vulnerability to pain. Zaniflex works on the sympathetic nervous system pathways in the brain. (Zaniflex is also said to reduce hot flashes on post-menopausal women, and has no estrogen hormone-like side effects.)

Zofran is a standard drug used to stop nausea for people taking cancer chemotherapy. It also blocks the release of substance P, a main neurochemical contributor to myofascial and fibromyalgia pain. Studies show that many people with fibromyalgia have improved by using Zofran.

The above medications, of course, can cause some side effects in some people, so see your doctor for any questions you may have.

Biochemistry and Metabolism

Since every body is very individual there are laboratories specializing in diagnosis that can help us detect metabolic imbalances and dysfunctions.

1. Essential fatty acid analysis which often shows a deficiency of omega-3 essential fatty acids. Certain amino acids analysis often shows a deficiency of the chain relationship of amino acids, with glutamine, taurine, tryptophan or tyrosine being the most common.

2. Other theories pertaining to alterations in neurotransmitters like serotonin and nor epinephrine. As mentioned before, substance P has an immune system function. Substance P is a pain neurotransmitter that has been found by repeat studies to be elevated three-fold in the spinal fluid of fibromyalgia patients. Two hormones that have been shown to be abnormal are cortisol and growth hormone (HGH).

3. A comprehensive digestive and stool analysis can point to digestive enzyme deficiencies, yeast, candida or Epstein-Barr, bacterial overgrowth, or even parasites, which most people will have. The key is your immune system can usually handle it and when it can't then you succumb to worse problems.
I feel that enhancing or strengthening the immune system is the best way to improve health with any disease.

4. Food allergies can be tested for as well or detected by going on an elimination diet. "Sensitive" food allergies can be identified that can make pain symptoms worse. Be careful with cleansing diets as I have found most people need building foods first due to poor eating habits. Urine tests for milk- or wheat-derived opioid peptides can pinpoint digestive abnormalities that lead to toxic by products. We have found most people are allergic to dairy products as well as to gluten found in wheat products. (See Dr. Andrew Weil's books on nutrition.) The key once again is that everybody is different and no fad diet can help everyone.

5. We used to do hair analysis or DMSA provoked urine testing to detect high levels of toxic metals like mercury or lead. Now we have many other systems for diagnosing and finding problems of that nature.

6. Checking the liver functions and enzyme levels is another way to find problems as the liver is a key organ for cleansing the body.

7. Ordering a screening T4/TSH is a good first approach as well. Many of the symptoms of fibromyalgia mimic hypothyroid muscular disease. Your doctor should order a screening thyroid test as part of the initial workup of fibromyalgia.

8. Checking for hyperthyroid is also done quite easily in the laboratory. Just make sure you are working with someone that takes the time to eliminate other potential problems that could appear as FMS.

Body-Therapy and Mind-Body Therapies

Great relief may come with just getting massage, however, it can also aggravate your condition so usually gentle massage is recommended and not deep tissue work. Many people with chronic muscle spasms or pain have tiny, taut fibrous bands or trigger points within the bellies or the origin and insertion of the muscles. These can be worked on with several techniques. One of the best techniques for these painful bands is DTF (Deep Transverse Friction), made popular by an orthopedic doctor from England named James Cyriax. He treated most of his patients with minor soft tissue injuries with this technique. With patients with fibromyalgia you have to be extremely careful to not create more irritation. You should see a professional massage therapist trained in this technique.

Trigger point therapy is another technique that helps reduce the stress in the tissues and also should be done with great care. As you will find, within these taut bands of muscle are extraordinarily sensitive pain points. These trigger points will help relieve the stress in the nervous system and also act to keep the entire muscle from having spasms. The problem with one muscle in spasm is that it puts its antagonist or assistant in stress too, and soon all the muscles are overtaxed in turn. This creates the muscle tug-of-war or a vicious cycle of muscle spasm, imbalance and pain, more tension, more pain, muscle imbalance, etc.

It takes professional knowledge to break this cycle. Sometimes just by balancing the pelvis, neck or back to allow the body proper mechanics will resolve the problem.. It may take heat or ice and DTF or trigger point therapy and gentle massage to turn it around. Other times it can take muscle relaxers or even cortosteroid injections. All of these can have value. The key is to know when to use or not use a specific treatment or medication. By injections we mean trigger point injections, or injections into ligaments or joints. These are called spinal facet joint injections, or epidurals. Sometimes acupuncture treatments can be beneficial along with the use of herbs. We mentioned massage and in that same area of body therapy techniques, we sometimes use mobilization or manipulations to free up the vertebrae or certain joints. These methods are used by osteopaths, chiropractors, and some manual therapists.

I said before that working to balance the hips or spine mechanics will often reduce the muscle tug-of-war, which then reduces the muscle-holding patterns in the body. These are some of the most effective treatments available to these patients. I have to keep telling the reader that it's critical to work with your doctor, and if he is not familiar with some of these natural modalities, share this article with him or her.

It's important to find highly qualified professionals, and just because you find a doctor it does not always mean he knows how to treat this condition. God only knows that the human body is a vast universe and no one person can know all there is about the body. That's why many of us in the medical fields have to specialize; by focusing on some aspect we get to understand it better. Then by working together we can assist all our patients better using the principles of synergy.

Most open minded doctors have found this to be true and have a vast network of health professionals to work in conjunction with, and for the betterment of, the patient.

Mind-Body Techniques

There is in the realm of body-mind techniques several that have proven effective in neurological balancing. The most popular and widely used are Traggering and Feldenkrais created by two extraordinary people who were pioneers in body-mind therapy. Milton Tragger was an M.D., a neurosurgeon who created a movement type of treatment that is gentle and achieves deep levels of relaxation through rocking motions. He was a friend and I got to know him in Honolulu and experience his work directly. We exchanged a few sessions with each other. It is very great, gentle system of work, soothing to the nervous system.

Feldenkrais was once associated with Ida Rolf, the mother of Rolfing. Rather than doing deep body work on the fasciae like Rolfing, Feldenkrais worked with certain body postures and movements to free up the patterns in the body since it often falls into poor posture and pain. Using movement and re-education of the body was his approach. His theory was to break up the neurological patterns of pain and restrictive movement.

Both of these techniques would be highly beneficial for people with fibromyalgia as they are gentle and would be very relaxing. They would assist in reducing the pain and tension at a structural neurological level. There are a few others that are similar: Aston patterning, Alexander Technique, and certain types of polarity therapy can all be helpful. Often it's not the technique as much as other factors. The most important aspect I have seen is the belief of the effectiveness of the therapy by the patient. In clinics that were set up for high volume injured patients, we knew that each individual responded differently to different treatments. There is no magic bullet in any medicine or in natural remedies. The key is to use what the patient feels more willing to follow, and then use the science of medicine and natural living to make it work for them.

It is funny how we could ever think of being in competition with anyone in the field of medicine. Heaven only knows there are plenty of sick and injured people out there. My biggest passion is to inspire people to the greatness of themselves, and to teach them about total health. We all know how important it is to our generation. It's been my focus my whole life; it's what I am about. Now after all these years, I have some understanding about applying all my knowledge of health to a real lifestyle that supports individuals on all levels of body, mind, and spirit.

More Mind Techniques

Of course, one of the best mental treatments for chronic pain and chronic illness, which takes a psychological toll on the mind as well as the body, is bio-feedback training, or some kind of relaxation or meditation techniques. These systems have been around for thousands of years, and only in their application do we think they are new. Almost everyone in the health field agrees that these are good techniques for pain. With stress being rampant in this modern day we could all benefit from learning how to relax without that after work martini.

There is a very useful technique call Neuro-Linguistic Programming or NLP, another mental tool that changes the physiology by focusing on a positive new pattern rather than on the old problem. And all of Tony Robinson's work is very powerful for transformations. I was lucky to have met him in the old days when I gave him a treatment and took all his seminars.

Just good old-fashioned deep breathing can do wonders for the pain and the stress level of any individual. Yoga and all the many forms of movement as we talked about before, tai chi or ballroom dancing, for anyone for that matter, may be helpful. The only advice I give in this area is never push or go into the pain, which will create the vicious cycle. Any endeavor we need to approach with some knowing and then take it easy.

Once again, all of the skills and tools mentioned above are available to us in our network of health professionals. Be sure and check with your doctor before trying some of the natural and holistic practices. Your health and well-being are what is most important.

What To Do If You Have FMS

In the long term, the most important thing you need to understand is that the first step is to understanding your fibromyalgia syndrome. We know that it can be chronic, but the symptoms or your episodes may flare up - or mellow out. This, we feel, can depend on your stress level, as well as what you have been doing to work on improving your condition. The impact that FMS has on daily living as well as activities is going to be different with each individual. It is commonly accepted that FMS can be as serious as rheumatoid arthritis in disabling people from working fulltime jobs. On the other hand, the chronic fatigue syndrome in CRS indicates that many people can improve. According to most experts, there are few that actually completely recover from it. I don't agree, and there are many new things coming up such as Hyper Immune Egg 26. There are not enough studies done on FMS yet to fully understand it.

Many patients have felt helpless or hopeless, and generally get very little relief or poor results. We must remember the best results come from using all the tools and methods available. It takes knowledgeable people as well as your commitment to becoming informed to begin getting better. Being in the health field most of my adult life, I know people with severe pain and frustration from having seen every doctor known to man, and it can get depressing or even suicidal with this disease or with severe back problems. Know that FMS is not a life-threatening disorder, although we can't say it's harmless. Some on the far end of the spectrum may feel like they can't live like this, but on the other side, some people can do well and live a good life.

Get your doctor to do the laboratory tests to rule out other possible maladies that can overlap or appear as FMS. One is hypothyroidism; it can be over-diagnosed but most commonly it's misdiagnosed. Fibromyalgia patients must have a good and thorough clinical diagnosis. Qualified medical doctors or osteopaths must make this diagnosis and ideally rule out other possibilities.

This disease can be confused with or be similar to MS (multiple sclerosis), lupus, osteoarthritis, rheumatoid arthritis, and even heart problems. You may have TMJ (temperomandibular joint syndrome), candida, Epstein-Barr syndrome, or CFS (chronic fatigue syndrome), or even Lou Gehrig's disease, a brain tumor, spine disease or a whole bunch of other problems. The only way to know it's FMS is to rule out some of these others, and only a qualified medical or osteopathic doctor can do this. Most clinical judgments are based on laboratory tests as well as the patient's history and a physical examination. You need to take the time to be clear that you do have FMS, and that the doctor making the diagnosis is experienced in it.

The best thing that we can suggest as health professionals is to find a doctor that you can work with that is open minded and can understand the complexity of working with this disorder. Using the information in this article and researching on the web at www.fibromyalgia.com or other sites that are similar will start to give you some hope to improve many of these symptoms. The key is that you have to take control of your own life and health.

Understand that to get better takes a whole lifestyle change and you need to understand what makes you better as well as what makes you worse. Sometimes it takes some experimentation as no human is the same and there is no magic pill.

You can start or join a FMS group. Also contact Fibromyalgia Network for a listing of patient contacts and physician referrals. The phone number is: (800) 853-2929. Other educational materials may be ordered from The Fibromyalgia Network Newsletter Resources.

May health be with you in all ways. . .

While we are at it we may as well look at its partner:

CHRONIC FATIGUE SYNDROME

First of all, I want to make it clear that this information is neither to diagnose nor to prescribe, and it should not take the place of the advice of your doctor. This is intended to complement conventional medicine, not to replace it. Consult with your doctor before starting any kind of nutritional or physical program.

Like fibromyalgia, CFS is rather hard to diagnose as it can have many ramifications as well as different causes. Let's take cause out of the equation and look at what the body could be telling us of how the person is living their life. In fact, often the two conditions are confused or found together. They have many similar symptoms as well, and I think the underlying weakness could be the immune system.

Also, as with fibromyalgia there are many symptoms including aching muscles or joints; anxiety; some depression or lack of concentration; poor appetite; sensitivity to infections and non-restorative sleep. Additionally, there are other sleep disorders like Periodic Leg Movement Disorder (PLMD),or sleep apnea, temporary memory loss, and most of all, extreme and sometimes disabling fatigue. Often there may be an inability for tolerating certain environmental factors such as stress, or even toxic metals may be present in the system. I feel many times the nutritional factors play a large role in a person's ability to cope with external factors.

Taking the first step of identifying these additional factors can give us a clearer picture of CFS to determine where to start, as more often than not there are many symptoms. Identifying these additional factors is crucial, since almost all of the separate symptoms have some type of treatment, yet often conventional drugs may not always work for the whole syndrome. Consequently, the more successful treatments use the holistic approach. This involves using conventional medical examinations and diagnosis with traditional treatments, and then including nutrition, herbs, and natural remedies as well as body/mind treatments like meditation, relaxation, imagery, and manual therapies like massage or acupuncture.

There are only a few centers in the United States that approach treatment in this fashion. We have so many medical centers and nutritional holistic centers, but few really integrate the two. One of the top centers is the Podell Medical Center in New Providence, New Jersey. It is one of the nation's leading centers for diagnosing and treating CFS as well as fibromyalgia and many other diseases. I really admire Dr. Podell's work. He is a medical doctor who looks at all the conventional medical approaches as well as natural methods for helping people, which is why they have so much success.

They are actually one of the few medical centers in the country using the holistic approach and they are using FDA approved phase III trials of the new drug for CFS, Ampligen.

As with fibromyalgia, one of the places Dr. Podell recommends starting with is nutrition.

Nutrition plays one of the key roles in all of health. Often yeast infections, or yeast candida and Epstein-Barr organisms preclude many of the diseases that we get because they feed on sugar in the system and they can only live in an acid environment. Excess meat and the lactose in dairy products contribute to creating an acid environment. It all breaks down to alcohol in the body. Looking at the body's blood sugar levels is a good place to start, with conventional medicine as well as nutritionally. Many people who suffer from this disorder may also have metal or mercury poisoning from dental work, or hypoglycemia, anemia, hypothyroidism, or even intestinal parasites. As I said before, there may be different combinations of factors contributing to the CFS. Medically we are not too sure what causes it, and it is said to not have a cure, even though many people do recover. Often it can re-occur with another illness or a heavy bout with stress. Treating "neurogenic hypertension," a low blood pressure syndrome that affects many people with CFS, by natural means including fluid, salt, potassium supplements, and licorice helps this condition. In a study at Johns Hopkins a connection was shown between CFS and regulating blood pressure. Patients with CFS who got lightheaded from long periods of standing benefited by treating the blood pressure problem.

Nutrition

Using the theory of alkaline balance that is recommended by Dr. Robert Young as nature's way to strengthen the immune system is a good place to begin. This can be achieved by reducing meat protein intake, sweets, and coffee while at the same time increasing green vegetables and perhaps finding a good green drink (chlorophyll is very important). Bringing the body back to an alkaline balance is one of the cornerstones to strengthening the immune system. Avoid shellfish, fried foods, junk food, soft drinks, and cut down on breads and pasta. Eat lots of garlic, or better yet, take (Kyolic) garlic in capsules that has been treated and has no odor.

Supplements

Very helpful for most of us for general well-being as well as anti-aging benefits are most anti-oxidant vitamins: Vitamin A 20,000 –30,000 IU daily; 10,000 - 20,000 IU's daily of natural beta carotene. Vitamin C, 5,000-10,000 mg daily (always take with bioflavanoids, buffered, an anti-viral and for strengthening the immune system); bromelain (Wobenzyme from Maryln Nutraceuticals), 1000 –3000 mg daily (Pineapple enzyme). I'm a great believer in this nutrient for many things. It is a natural anti-inflammatory nutrient that reduces inflammation, not only in the joints but it also works on the tissues. Vitamin E, 400-800 IU; Also pycnogenol or grape seed extract, both anti-inflammatory and anti-oxidant; magnesium, 500-1,000 mg; Manganese, 5 mg daily; Vitamin D, 500 IU daily. N-Acetyl Cysteine, 500-1000 mg. This nutrient is converted in the body to glutathione. It has definite mucous-thinning and anti-oxidant effects. Supplements including essential fatty acids, L-Carnitine, Coenzyme Q-10, 75 mg daily; glutathione precursors and acidophilus capsules (to renew the friendly bacteria in the system). Also, very important would be free-form amino acid complex as they assist in tissue and organ repair.

Injections

Vitamin B complex, 2 cc injections twice weekly or as prescribed by your physician. Vitamin B-6, 1/2 cc twice weekly or as prescribed; B-12, 1 cc twice weekly or as prescribed; Niacin (vitamin B-3) or niacinamide. If injections are not available liver extract can be beneficial or Vitamin B complex, 100 mg 3 times a day, plus extra B-12, 2,000 mcg daily. Sublingual form is best for most vitamins. (See Dr. Robert Young on the web.)

Glandular Therapy

Some physicians that work with nutrition also recommend raw thymus, spleen, and raw glandular complex.

Herbs

Herbs are not to be used daily; they should only be used during heavy bouts.
Licorice, black currant or primrose oil supply essential fatty acids. Milk thistle, St. John's wort, ginseng, ginkgo biloba, comfrey, and kava (Hawaiian kava-kava). Creatine can help as well. A tea brewed with burdock root, dandelion and red clover promotes healing by

cleansing the blood and enhancing the immune function. There, of course, are many mushrooms available now for strengthening the immune system. Use shitake, the most common, also, reishi and mitake. Eat these with your meals or use capsules purchased in health food stores.

Sleep Therapy

Meditation and relaxation training increase the resistance to stress. Using biofeedback, imagery, self-hypnosis, and spiritual values can all help for increased wellness as well as sleep improvement. Some of the amino acids taken for nutrition will help sleep. Extra melatonin could also be helpful for more restful sleep. Scullcap and valerian root can aid in sleep. Always use caution with herbs.

MANUAL THERAPY

Massage is becoming a much more accepted treatment for many medical problems. Not only does it help with circulatory problems, it also has more far reaching effects than most people realize by healing through the release of histamines and hormones. In specific DTF (deep transverse friction) invented by Dr. James Cyriax, it can alleviate pain, reduce inflammation and break up adhesions. All forms of massage must be done specifically for intended results and care must be taken for fibromyalgia patients as it could make conditions worse, so consult a professional. Structural evaluation and that type of work can also be very beneficial, especially to reduce structural stress on the body. Even a gentle exercise program can have great benefit. Care must be used in all of these therapies.

Acupuncture may be helpful for some of these conditions when we don't have clear and understandable symptoms. It assists the body in strengthening itself and does not usually work on attacking a specific disease.

Finally, to get the best of all worlds, we seek an integrated approach for all illness, as well as for wellness.

Sources: Most of this work was taken from Dr. Podell who has a clinic for the treatment of fibromyalgia, as well as the works of Hans C. Hansen; Dr.Pellegrino, M.D., Ohio State University in 1989; The Rheumatic Disease Clinics of North America (22(2):219-243, 1996), and Debra Buchwald, M.D.

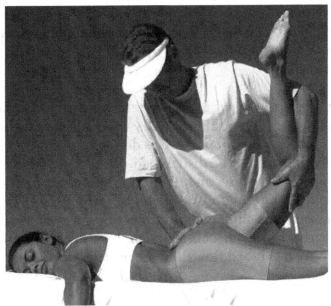

CHAPTER THREE
BODY PARTS

As we have said before, our belief structures sometimes get in the way. We need to look at the physical structure, real flesh and blood. To study the body from a structural point of view, let's start with the muscles.

Muscles

Muscles consist mostly of water and are the motors that move every part of the body. You can't talk, walk, breathe, eat or drink without using muscles. They all produce movement by the same method, contraction. They pull on their tendons or attachments, which in turn move the levers (the bones). For example, when the biceps (on the front of your upper arm) contracts, the forearm and hand are brought toward your body. Then to extend the arm away you must contract the opposing muscle, the triceps.

They are symbolic of our motivation in life; they move us. They build fast and heal fast as they have a large blood supply moving though them, which you can tell by their bright red color. We will cover the major muscles in great detail later in this book, as I believe that understanding muscles is vital for training and fitness, and most of all for therapy.

Tendons

Tendons are strong, fibrous bands that attach muscles to bone; they are not flexible like muscle. Muscles and tendons are very similar, differing only slightly in composition and cell structure. Tendons are rope-like extensions of the muscles, but they don't contract; only muscle cells do that.

To understand better what a tendon is, find the wide part of your calf muscle in the middle part of the back of your lower leg. The tendon starts where the wide calf muscle suddenly becomes a narrow band above your heel. This is the Achilles tendon. With your hand, follow the band down to where it attaches to the back of your heel bone. Notice that when the calf muscle contracts, it pulls the Achilles tendon up, which in turn pulls the front part of the foot down (in plantar flexion).

When muscles are shortened by hard exercise, tension in the muscle-tendon complex is increased. Tendons are more susceptible to injury than muscles are for two reasons. First, tendons have a smaller cross section than muscles do. That means they don't have as large or as wide an area over which force can be distributed. As a result, exercise typically puts more strain on tendons than on muscles. Second, tendons are located in areas where they can be injured easily, usually at the origin and insertion of the muscles. They are located at the attachment points and some have no sheath or protection. In contrast, muscles are located in protected areas. They rarely rub against other rough tissue. Tendons take longer to build and longer to heal, as they have less blood flow than the muscles do.

Joints and Cartilage

A joint is the place between two bones that functions like a hinge so that the bones can move in relation to each other. Some joints have minimal movement, like the ribs, skull bones and the spine, when compared to others, like the shoulder or knee.

Cartilage is a tough, white gristle structure, the shock absorber between bones. This tissue contains few blood vessels or nerves. It covers the ends of the bones of a joint to prevent the bones from rubbing against each other. If cartilage is torn, broken, or chipped, the end of the bone is unprotected and gradually can irritate the whole area from the friction against the cartilage of the opposing bone. Movement will become painful because the end of the exposed bone contains a rich supply of nerves. A common injury is cartilage damage to the knees, often called "torn cartilage." It can result from "hits" as in football and other sports, or from twists to the knees, or with falls, skiing, skating, etc. Knee injuries are only second to ankle injuries as the most common sports injuries.

Ligaments

Ligaments are tough, fibrous bands that attach to the ends of bones where they meet to form a joint. Their main function is to hold the bones together when the joint moves. They are not at all flexible and have very little blood supply, so they are very slow to heal (and consequently, long to build as well). Ligaments can hold the bones together so tightly as to restrict the movement of the joint. Like the vertebrae in your spine, ligaments can move only slightly, but can also be flexible enough to allow a wide range of motion. The best example of the most mobile joint is the shoulder. Consider all the movement possible in the hips, knees, ankles, toes, elbows, wrists and fingers, for these joints are all held together with ligaments, as well as muscles.

Injuries

All joint injuries, whether they involve bones, cartilage, ligaments, or the muscles and tendons that attach near the joint, have the potential to end an athletic career, be it professional or recreational.

If some of the fibers of the ligament are torn, it is called a sprain. To avoid further tearing of these fibers, the joint should be immobilized immediately. No stretching -- it's amazing that our coaches always said to "run it off or stretch"! This is often the worst thing to do for a strain (muscle), or sprain (ligament), as that pulls the injury farther apart. Of course, RICE will help (Rest, Ice, Compression and Elevation). If all of the fibers are torn, the injury is called a complete ligamentus rupture. In most cases, the ligament reattaches itself by laying down new cells, but if the tear is severe, surgery may be needed. Most sprains, however, can be helped with DTF (Deep Transverse Friction), a very specific form of massage, and RICE.

Treatment and Healing

If you incur an injury to any joint, whether it is your shoulder, elbow, wrist, fingers, hip, knee, ankle or toe, treat it immediately with RICE. Never exercise or stretch a joint that has just been injured. If the pain or swelling is severe or lasts beyond 48 hours, seek help from a sports medicine doctor. I realize that in most cases the pain will not be gone in 48 hours, and as a result many people may see their doctors unnecessarily. However, the diagnosis and management of joint injury requires special training that cannot be taught in a book. So, it's safer to send you to a doctor needlessly than to take the chance that you won't receive the proper diagnosis and treatment for a potentially serious problem.

A ligament that is over stretched results in pain, just as other over-stretched tissues do. Even the muscles can be torn and need treatment. Ligaments will hurt more with passive movement and ROM (range of motion) of the injured area. Often ligaments will hurt under weight-bearing or just walking. The pain associated with an over-stretched ligament is sharp and seems to be more localized than in muscle injuries. The affected area may feel either hot or cold, or it may feel like a tearing sensation.

DTF and Healing

While healing, the ligament can adhere to adjacent muscle or bone, decreasing mobility as well as increasing future injuries. DTF (Deep Transverse Friction) shifts the ligament in imitation of its natural movement and prevents it from adhering to adjacent muscle and bone. In fact, DTF aids all adhesions whether they are new (acute) or old (chronic). Old injuries just take longer; acute injuries heal much faster with DTF. Ice combined with DTF can be used effectively for the first week to ten days, and much longer thereafter, but NO HEAT. You should NEVER apply heat to injuries (even after 48 hours, especially if there is still pain). Heat should only be used for muscle tension or women's menstrual cramps, as it brings blood to the surface muscles to help them relax. Ice, however, brings blood deep into the tissues; it is an analgesic as well as an anti-inflammatory aid. Ice is some of the best medicine available to us. Actually water in general is a great healer, in all its forms, from just swimming in the ocean to showers, steam baths, hot mineral baths, to ice. It is very healing.

Fascia (Connective Tissue)

Fasciae are the thick or at times thin, white, fibrous sheets that surround, protect, and support almost all the tissue in the body, including muscles, tendons, joints, nerves, blood vessels and organs. Fascia looks and feels somewhat like ligaments and tendons, and contains the same four components: two types of fibers, fluid and connective tissue cells. In athletes, fasciae absorb some of the pressure on tendons, muscles, and joints, protecting them from injury or too much movement. Fascia is not very flexible, nor does it heal quickly. It can be very hard in some areas, almost sticking organs or muscles together. These adhesions can be a sign of stress or injury to the tissue. There is not a lot of blood flow through fascia, and it is slow to change.

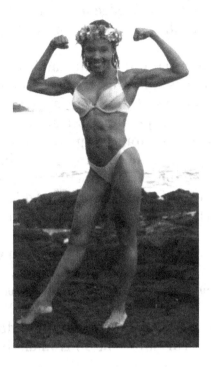

CHAPTER FOUR
The Laws of Training

There are so many stories concerning sports and training. In the old days, I heard of one guy picking up his calf every day, and as the calf got bigger he got stronger. It's kind of funny, but that is actually one of the laws of training called "Adaptability" -- the body will adapt to the stress that you put on it. Ancient mythology had funny ways of putting things then. It's difficult to know what really works in sports, but one key for me is to use the knowledge that the ancient people used. After all, much "folk medicine" goes back thousands of years, as does Chinese medicine, Ayurvedic medicine, all the tribal knowledge of herbs and the importance of the spirit in healing as well as living. We could use more of that good old-fashioned medicine even now. Oddly, using these traditional approaches with modern medicine is now called "integrative" ("holistic" is out), but allopathic medicine is only a few hundred years old. I think we could learn much from the old medicine. The best approach is using the old with the new, if I may be so bold...

I don't know if you followed news of health and fitness over the years, but back in the fifties and sixties we were far behind the East Germans and Russians in athletics and sports medicine. For most people, it was hard to get research papers on sports medicine or training back then. Knowledge in this field was mostly reserved for the elite, professional athletes.

We now can hold our own in world competition. We have learned a lot more about sports medicine since that time, and we are also more aware of what is mistakenly called "alternative medicine." I think that allopathic medicine is the actual "alternative." Natural healing methods and what we call folk medicine are thousands of years old. Anyway, why not work together? Those of us who think it is more fun to work together would rather call it "integrative medicine" if it's medicine at all. However, I believe all the disciplines need to work together, to get the most out of knowledge in sports medicine for the betterment of all bodies. Besides, the Hippocratic Oath is "first, do no harm."

We used to think that there were natural athletes and there were limitations to certain performances. Having good genetics still holds true. The Eastern Europeans used to biopsy the muscle tissue of the athletes to see if they had fast-twitch or slow-twitch muscle. Fast-twitch muscle favors sprinters and quick-action athletes. Slow-twitch muscle can be developed for intense strength and endurance-type athletes. We have since found that you can modify the muscle type by scientific training. They, however, guided their athletes towards the sport that most suited their muscle twitch. This was one reason why they were getting better results with many of their athletes. Added to that, they were worked specifically for their sport, which made them even more successful.

In the seventies and eighties, many runners would run up to 90 miles a week, always at the same pace. They didn't know about specificity in training, which meant just that. If they didn't train at the speed they wanted to compete in, they would not achieve that speed in competition, or at least not good enough to be using their full abilities. Many of the athletes now know the five laws of training. For those of you who don't, I will go over them. Why should the pros have all the fun? This information is valuable to anybody who is looking to get fit.

As a therapist in a renowned clinic in LA from 1975 to 1977, I got to work with some of the top sports medicine chiropractors who used Kinesiology in their practice. Dr. John Thie and Dr. Leroy Perry were among the most highly regarded chiropractors working with many top athletes at that time. Perry was working with some of the Olympic athletes, however, because of politics, we could not use all the knowledge available to us for our Olympic athletes in their sports training. We need to start cooperating and working together, to get the most out of our systems. Not everyone has all the tools or the answers, in fact, the longer I'm in the business the more it sometimes seems that there are no answers, other than to just live you life.

In Russia they were using all the physical, natural, scientific, and new age technologies they could get their hands on for training their athletes. They were biopsing athletes' muscles, they were using drugs, hormone enhancers, nutrition, sports psychology and who knows what else.

Eastern European and Russian athletes were dominating most international sports, so quite arguably they were doing something right. Sometime later it was obvious that there was negative impact on many of their athletes; their careers were intense but often short. They seemed to get old fast and who knows what else they went through in terms of pain and suffering. World competition athletics is a very powerful arena to walk into. Just think about it: In some way all of us are athletes, we all have certain physical and mental demands. Well, they are all self-imposed, of course, but there, nonetheless. Training for the sake of training is more powerful than stressing yourself to train to help you with your daily stress. You know what I mean: Think of that man down the street that jogs every day, but when you pass him he looks like it's hell and he is not enjoying it. But he thinks it's going to help him to be healthy, and by god, he's going to force himself to run even if it kills him.

The difference is that you have to enjoy life first! Then all the other things we do are just us doing life. In Europe there was a very high respect for tradition and for each person as an individual. The main thing was they put egos aside and did the best they could for the athletes, as far as they knew at the time. We are learning more about fitness every day.

In training at the level of a statewide track and field team of elite Nike Runners, we knew that without the cutting edge science of sports medicine available, our athletes couldn't keep up in racing events. To heighten performance, I used structural massage, made specific muscle evaluations, and prescribed specific muscle improvement exercises for our team. We tested nutritional eating plans using nurturing foods, power foods, raw juices, and natural minerals, and we included blue-green algae, bee pollen, ginseng, and dong quai among other things. I had been experimenting with foods and eating plans since 1969, and had been studying nutrition, herbology, fasting, wild edible plants, and Native American healing methods. We now know the importance of what we eat and how it contributes directly to the body/mind and its performance. Well, at least most of us do.

By the time I hit Hawaii way back in 1977, I had been on the training and therapy path for ten years (still a babe in some circles), yet I felt I was just beginning to grasp some new concepts. At the time, the old style training methods and thinking prevailed. Many doctors said that it didn't matter what you ate. Many athletes were just out there training hard and often and sustaining many injuries. No systems to speak of, although there were a few athletes I'd met who kept very detailed records and they did train better and differently than most. However, these individuals were few and far between. You see, these were people doing an intuitive training program and some of them were very successful at achieving many of their fitness and competitive goals. Most, however, were out there running in space and were spaced out running.

In 1983 the Outrigger Canoe Club of Honolulu would actually eat steak and potatoes the night before their grueling 26-mile race from Molokai to Oahu. They were only lifting weights, very heavy all the time. At times these races go on in 10 to 15 foot seas, and they are extremely demanding. Many traditional trainers had different views and techniques or modalities concerning how to train for this event. Many of the new techniques were different and many were out of their realm of expertise. They were not too open to some of the new methods of training. Massage, nutrition, sports imagery, and the holistic approach were very definitely not the norm in the early to mid 1970s, and still now in 2004.

We taught our team about carbo-loading and specificity in training. Before loading you must carbo-starve by increasing protein during hard training. The Russian athletes of 1976 used all the most advanced training methods to date. Nutrition in America was still considered very subjective or vague in its true applications to sports and competition.

In 1984 when we first started working with the Outrigger Canoe Team, we started with weight training and used specificity in the action needed for paddling, along with nutrition, imagery and other new age methods. Some of these big jocks would just laugh at us, they would giggle while we were using some NLP (Neuro-Linguistic Programming) and imagery with creative visualizations to teach them how to relax and improve focus. These were not new then but we had never really had the opportunity to totally apply everything that I had been studying and using on myself. Here was my second chance with a big time team and we had carte blanche to do whatever we thought would work to train them for this great race.

Then as now, many athletes don't know very much about total body-mind training. Some of the biggest weightlifters I would work with would laugh at my small 195 lb, 6'2" frame and say "you're the muscle man?" (This is what some of the jocks called me.) It was because of my work in Kinesiology that they called me "the muscle man," not because I had them, well, at least not huge one; mine were just right for me.

Many of these athletes as well as weightlifters were big guys and the only other person they respected or listened to was someone bigger and stronger than they were. It's a real macho environment full of testosterone. What's funny is that I've worked with a lot of female teams, too, and the women are just as intense, pardon me, ladies, if not more intense. Athletes are just in a human category all by themselves.

Now more athletes are interested in the science of training and many of the new approaches of holistic or integrative medicine. Training today is so scientific that an athlete, trainer, or coach who fails to understand the power of science and teamwork, or who doesn't stay informed about the latest training discoveries, will not be able to keep up. Wow, what pressure, but it's true. In the Olympic to professional levels the pressure to perform at the top of your ability is intense for everyone involved, from the athlete to the coaches, the trainers and even the families connected with it all. Athletes, coaches, and trainers all suffer at the high levels of competition, but that's the nature of the beast. It's push, push, push and there is a lot of pressure to perform. Not asking for help during these times is a way to get lost on the way to the forum. We need to look at all the factors of training if we are to excel in any sport or to be totally fit for that matter.

Back in the '70s and '80s only the professional or Olympic athletes were able to take advantage of the latest scientific information and therapies. It was not readily available to most of us weekend warriors. We need to acknowledge that there are certain immutable laws in training and no one is above these laws.

Let's Look at the Laws of Training:

1) **Specificity**
2) **Hard & Easy Days**
3) **Training & Rest**
4) **Base & Peaking**
5) **Reversibility**

1) Specificity

Specificity is one of the laws of training we can't avoid. To perfect a sport or skill, you must practice using your muscles in the same manner you would during the specific activity. Your training must be very specific, well, that sounds logical. Lifting weights over your head will not make you paddle harder, stronger or better. Those guys in the Outrigger Canoe Team were all bulking up by lifting weights just to get strong, but their exercise regime was not specific enough for the paddling action they needed to improve most. To remedy that they rigged up pulley systems for specific action in the paddle stroke. That made a lot of difference in how we could improve performance.

You also need to train at the level you intend to compete in. Running ten-minute miles will not help you compete at four-minute miles. Many runners were not doing speed drills, nor were they doing enough interval training for their specific needs to improve their running ability in speed. Because you can't always train at full speed either, they were lost about having a system that would do both, but that will bring us to a few more laws.

Also, we must consider what kind of body we have to work with because genetics plays a very important part in athletic success. Some bodies are predisposed for certain physical perfection and skills. I believe there are natural born athletes. I've met many who possessed great gifts of natural strength, speed and endurance. The main thing is what you do with your gift once you recognize it. The type of training you select could make the difference between a good athlete and a great athlete. Nowadays, to be competitive in the world of sports most athletes have to be naturally gifted to start with, and then train specifically to get better and become great.

Whatever physical training we undertake, for whatever reason, we need to define where we are and where we intend to go.

In my opinion, full muscle and joint evaluation should be done for each person to know exactly which muscles he or she needs to work with. Most bodies have misalignments in the bones, vertebrae or pelvis, as well as among the muscles. We have all fallen and suffered injuries, or have genetic predispositions to some structural challenges. We have all inherited some of our parents' strengths as well as their weaknesses. Genetic predisposition has positive and negative impact in how it can affect us. We all have muscles that are too weak or too strong, too loose or too tight. Believe me, even super powerful athletes have some relative muscle imbalances and weaknesses. In my opinion achieving postural and muscular balance is key to a fully working physical body. Then it can work at full capacity. So to build a body, I believe that we should begin work with a well balanced body, and not build on the body's imbalances.

Structure governs function. The more balance and true strength the athlete has, the more efficiently that body will operate. It's all about mechanics and physics, science, not philosophy or a belief structure -- well maybe, but that's another book. Once the weak or tight muscles are identified, it's much easier in training to use the proper exercises for that particular body, not only for strengthening but for stretching and fine tuning as well. Knowing which muscles need specific exercise prevents many unnecessary hours of skewed workouts which only underscore present imbalances.

It is very important to build the body in, and with, balance. This prevents the stress that arises when opposing muscles get neglected. It can also create an unstable joint. This muscle tug-of-war can cause over use of muscles, promote inefficiency in movement, possibly create injuries down the road, and waste energy if the balance is not efficiently correct.

Using the science of sports medicine, Kinesiology, exercise physiology, biochemistry, and other natural healing and training methods, we are able to help almost anyone keep the body and muscles in balance as they build. By using massage, corrective balance restoring exercises, specific strength training, Pilates, yoga, acupressure and manipulations, we can create a finely tuned human machine with increased flexibility, strength and range of movement.

2. Hard and Easy Days

Some exercise enthusiasts get addicted to working out and over training can become a problem, usually for the elite athletes. For the body to improve, it's critical that it have time to recuperate and heal as well. You need to schedule hard days for intensive workouts, interspersed with easy days for recovery. Resting is just as important as fatiguing the muscles in order to build strength or endurance. This is also known as irritability and adaptability. Professional athletes don't perform the same workout each day and neither should you. When I first started working with some of the top runners in Hawaii, I was amazed at how many miles they were putting in. Some were doing between 80 to 100 miles a week - yes, *a week*, I said.

You don't need that much quantity once you have a base, unless you are training to be a marathon runner. "LSD (Long Slow Distance) is way out." I would say "just let me hit your legs with a 2 x 4 and then run 30 miles less; you'll get the same benefit." In serious athletic training, it's good to get your heart rate up to 80 or 90 percent of your maximum every day, but my god, you don't need to pound the pavement for that many miles.

You need slow and long only for building the base. Once it is built very few slow workouts are necessary. That is, unless you just want basic fitness, however, for competitive racing you need more high-intensity for peaking and speed training for your finishes.

I suggested that they vary the workouts and follow the hard-easy principle. Cross training started to make some headway during those days. I found that the easy days could be cycling, swimming or weight training. But if you want to be the best of the best, then specificity is the answer and cross training is out. This has to be more scientific, and the more focused, and the better results will come from it.

2a) Hard Days

Hard days are those when you put nearly 100% into your workout. Improvement comes from these hard days when the body is stressed and you push it even further to the next level. Protein becomes important as it repairs damaged tissue. Minerals and water are crucial nutritional elements at this level of training and also become more critical since muscles require all of them in order to function at optimum levels. Often it's on these days that we suffer micro-trauma to the muscles, which creates a sore feeling the day after. Minor muscle tears do occur, and you may notice in some weightlifters those muscle tears become big bumps. For a performance athlete these need time to repair to function at their best, or else you have scar tissue and ineffective muscle function.

Stress refers to the intensity an athlete puts into the workout, not necessarily the amount of time spent working out. The body must be stressed for a specific and increased amount of time in order to safely improve and strengthen. Irritation and adaptability is a fine line. The time will vary with the sport and your condition, but usually the exercise must be intense enough to make you breathe harder, sweat, and increase your heart rate. Of course, care must be taken in this stress-and-heal activity to avoid tearing down what has been so carefully built.

As beginners, most runners are told to not go too fast and that they should be able to hold a conversation as they jog. Of course, this is to build a base, because if you start panting so that you can't breathe you're not going to exercise your body long enough to enjoy a decent workout. Plus you go into oxygen debt and don't improve much or burn fat, and you can get hurt if you go too far. The beginner's pulse could go over 60-70% of their maximum heat rate to improve. You've all seen those charts that have you subtract your age from 220 to calculate your maximum heart rate. To attain the level of a trained athlete you need to reach 90% of your maximum and sustain that level for 60 to 90 minutes or longer, depending on the sport.

One way to calculate your training level is to subtract your age from the number 220; that number is your maximum heart rate. Most coaches recommend to start training at about 60% of your maximum, and to increase monthly by three to five percent until ultimately you train near 90% of your maximum heart rate (see building a base). Then, to find your training level, multiply your maximum by 60 or 70%.

Age	Maximum heart rate	Heart training rate
Beginner (training baseline)		
20	220 - 20	= 200 x 60% = 120 training rate
50 and over	220 - 50	= 170 x 60% = 102 training rate
Fit athlete		
20	220 – 20	= 200 x 90% = 180 training rate
40	220 – 40	= 180 x 90% = 162 training rate

2b) Easy Days

As we said, stressing the body for competition and hard training causes minor injuries to muscles that require time to heal (see section on micro trauma). That's why we need massage as well, not only rest, and also some easy workouts. We turned these into fun days of training.

For example, we played the "rabbit and the hounds" game. A rabbit (fast runner) would run out ahead of the pack (us dogs) and leave clues for us to find. We would use ribbons, paint, food or funny undergarments. Anyway, you get the picture. The point was that we got a hell of a workout chasing the rabbit while trying to be the first team to collect the clues and find the rabbit's hideout, because that's where the food and beer were waiting for us to enjoy after training. Beer is great stuff for training. (All in moderation.)

That's why you must work easy days into your training program; the body needs to recover or you will enter a tear down cycle (Selye). Instead of running every day but one, some runners started to do an easy run combined with a hard swim or bike. This would keep their heart working yet give their legs and feet a break from pounding the pavement. I think this is how cross training was born. I always had athletes do alternative training when they were hurt to keep the heart rate level of fitness because that is what is lost first. Some would swim with drag floaters and just use their arms if their legs were hurt. I would sometimes have them use a bike with their hands to keep up that heart rate.

Recovery Time

You will benefit from a heavy workout only if you allow your muscles time to recover. If your muscles are stressed again before that happens, they deteriorate and you will lose ground. I have seen some runners really suffer because they never relaxed long enough to allow for muscular recuperation time. There are signs of Over Training. Many elite athletes experience excessive weight loss, fatigue, and pain in the feet, ankles, knees, hips, low back, upper back, and even pain in the neck and butt. Under major stress, it's the weakest skeletal link that breaks down. I really believe that, and the tightest muscles usually are the ones that suffer most. That means if you start running and your hip is out of balance, or your neck is out of alignment you will experience worse symptoms in those places. I've always said to my patients to just start running and you will find out where your weak link is. Running will bring out the worst in all of us! For those of you that don't need to run, walking is great and can get you fit without the aches and pains. To really get fit, however, running is the best all around way to get fit the fastest.

Muscle fibers are damaged by hard workouts, which cause micro-traumas, those nagging little aches and pains we athletes have endured forever. Until sports massage came along, many athletes just thought it was a normal part of life to have those pains. Like any other tissue in the body, muscle requires healing time proportionate to the amount of stress withstood or inflicted on it. Of course, we all know that people heal at different rates due to their genetic predisposition, body type, attitude about life and age. A recovery period or an easy day does not mean we do nothing. We must still work out, at least for the cardiovascular aspect, but less intensely on other parts of the body. Performing at a relaxed pace hastens recovery more than doing nothing.

Remember we talked about cross training? I've always found that swimming or bicycling after a running event helps to keep the body from getting stiff. Recovery from competition usually takes even longer than recovery from a heavy workout. There are many factors for this because as we get caught up in the excitement of the race we go beyond our normal bounds and suffer later.

Professional football teams have also adopted the hard-easy technique. Sunday usually is game day, their hardest day. On Monday the players review game films, soak in the tub, get treated for injuries, do stretching exercises and run a light drill to work up a sweat; basically, they take it easy. Tuesday is a day off for most players unless they need rehabilitation. Then many get massage, PT work or other rehabilitation work. Wednesday is game plan day with the most physically challenging practice of the week where they train at 70-90% of their cardiac maximum. They run their plays and have their most intense workout of the week. There's a moderately hard workout on Thursday and a very easy day on Friday, consisting mostly of easy runs and a flexibility workout, maybe some more therapy and soaking. On Saturday players polish up their game plan and travel if the game is out of town. Sunday is back to all out football. They normally don't lift weights once the season has started; most of them bulk up during off season. So it's mostly an easy and hard day type of program during the regular season.

They know the importance of peaking too. Many NFL teams have included more stretching in their regime now that they know it helps to prevent injury and improve speed.

Coaches and athletes have debated for years about the optimum recovery period. Even now coaches can't agree on the proper interval of time between hard workouts. With most athletes I've worked with we recommended a 48-hour recovery period from hard workouts, games or competitions.

3) Training and Rest

Athletes who have extended the frontiers of the human body by prodigiously increasing its workload have brought about the fantastic improvement in athletic performance over the last 25 years. Athletes are now routinely doing things that were assumed to be beyond our human capacity just a few decades ago, like breaking the four-minute mile. Percy Cerutty, an Australian running coach who employs very unusual methods in training his runners, was responsible for training the athletes that broke some of these records. He used animal style running and jumping to strengthen muscles (more about this in the running section) along with modified gaits, and lifting the arms while running to increase oxygen intake. There have been many types of discoveries in training and we are discovering more every day. This human body is something amazing. I think if you look at where the human body has come since we were cavemen, we realize the miracle. High school athletes are currently obliterating swimming and some running and jumping records of the '80s and '90s. Every year we see more touchdowns, yards and baskets in all the sports. We are moving forward at an awesome rate, but to what extent does this help the rest of us who just want to be fit and healthy? We are training at much more intense levels, and this gives us all the more reason to keep in mind the rest factor.

Over Training

There is a limit to the amount of work even the most highly conditioned athlete should undertake. There's a fine line between work and building, and overwork and destroying. I know a few intense athletes who over trained themselves out of great careers. There are too many I know who sustained minor injuries, refused to rest and did not permit the body to heal, making their injuries worse.

Many careers have been ended by injury before athletes win an Olympic medal, or even break their personal record, or just win that state 10K. I know, I was one of these crazy guys, and more than that, I've treated hundreds of these athletes driven to succeed in competition as well as with their own Type A personality at training. Many can't compete anymore because they didn't recognize the signs of Over Training.

Dr. Seyle on Stress and Over Training

Dr. Hans Selye, the physician from Montreal who coined the word "STRESS," conducted a famous experiment that showed if rats were stressed and then allowed to recover, they became stronger. Rats that were stressed again before they recovered became weaker. Rats that were not stressed didn't improve in health, strength or conditioning. And something controversial: They didn't get smarter. I learned about Dr. Selye's work on stress and over training in a seminar I took in the early '70s in California. I got a chance to meet and talk with him personally. I bought his book 20 years ago and still have it. In it he describes some of the symptoms of over training which include always feeling tired, suffering from frequent colds and injuries, and experiencing nagging aches and pain.

Here are the more specific signs of Over Training:

Muscular Symptoms of Over Training

Symptoms include persistent soreness and stiffness in the muscles, joints, and tendons. Your feet may hurt and you may feel heavy-legged. Everything hurts until you start running again, and then you feel better until you stop and feel your body a few hours later. Night cramps are common, but severe night cramps are also a symptom of deficiency in electrolytes or from not drinking enough water.

The muscles ache daily, even on easy days, due to micro-trauma. There are little tears to the minute muscle fibers, which have been strained during excessive workouts. Without enough time to heal they cry out with pain. Little knots pop up on many areas and when you massage them, they hurt. You know -- I'm sure you have a few somewhere.

Emotional Symptoms

Athletes who are over training sometimes find it hard to get going in the morning and may experience a loss of interest in training. THIS IS WEIRD! This can be accompanied by unexplained nervousness, uneasiness, and an inability to relax. I have even noticed depression in some of these athletes due to lost races or missed opportunities. Many go into denial about their troubles. You need to be aware of all these aspects if you are working with some of these athletes who are constantly on edge. Under these circumstances, a drop in academic or work performance is not uncommon, and sometimes, in order to recover, a dependency on drugs or liquor starts to form.

Warning Signs of Over Training

Other symptoms of over training include frequent headaches, loss of appetite, and a sudden drop in athletic performance. Body and mind fatigue, sluggishness and a general feeling that you have "hit a wall" all come up. Sometimes we see swelling of muscles, joints, and of lymph nodes in the neck, groin or armpit. Infections can develop from blisters or other cuts; they just don't seem to heal well. Any type of constipation or diarrhea could get out of hand during this episode. Some weight loss is not uncommon in long distance runners, but too much weight loss or loss in body fat can be dangerous, especially for women. Many female athletes experience adverse changes in the menstruation cycle, or a suspension of it altogether (amenorrhea) when they over train. Often we see women athletes who lose their breasts and become stressed in many other ways.

Over training is a serious problem among beginners, amateurs and even some elite athletes. Beginners who don't take the time to build a proper base can do too-much-too-soon for their poorly conditioned and out of shape bodies to handle. They then can become injured or fatigued and quit their program. Seasoned elite, amateur, and professional athletes who overwork are all frequently injured and often dragging. The result is less than their best performance. I think everyone I know has "hit the wall" at some point in their athletic career, especially the driven ones. The key is to know how to get out of it without serious injury and how to get back on the track.

For many years the coaches relied on athletes to tell them how they felt to determine if they were Over Training. If the athlete reported feeling fine, they were free to train -- not very scientific, but generally it worked OK. For the more elite or professional athletes this may not work, because they'll rarely say they are not OK. They have come so far that many of them just live with pain, especially if we are talking about football or other contact sports. They are used to it and often think that's just part of the game.

The other common method for determining your state is to measure the resting pulse rate. If it's more than six or seven beats per minute above normal, the athlete should take the day off, so an easy workout is recommended. European trainers take blood samples from their athletes to check for blood enzyme concentration, or for an increase in the red blood cell count, both of which indicate that the body is stressed and needs to recover.

All in all, well-trained athletes should know when they are doing too much. Otherwise, they should work with coaches and trainers who are educated to know when their athletes are training too much and correct the situation.

Guard Against Over Training

To improve maximally, you must increase your body's capacity by increasing its workload, but not by going beyond its limits. This is a fine line to tread in training. Massage and corrective alignment exercises boost the body's capability for recovery. Eating the right foods and getting the proper amount of rest is the remainder of the equation. Learning the proper systems of training becomes a key factor in athletic performance. Keeping the awareness growing as you get in better shape will show in your increased abilities. We must realize one thing: The higher the level of competition you get to, the more important everything you do becomes, and the less improvement you get. Each gain is more difficult. That's why it literally becomes a science to get the most out of training for ultimate performance.

4) Building the Base and Peaking

Your training should begin with laying a foundation upon which you progressively increase your workload and its duration. You can prepare the body for future stress with high intensity workouts, and longer endurance building sessions later. The base is critical for fortifying the infrastructure of muscle, tendon, ligaments, and bones.

Athletes who compete in endurance events must learn to alternate between base and peaking. A month before competition, the athlete should start decreasing the volume and increasing the intensity of the workouts, making sure to get plenty of rest and fluids, then follow with the carbo-starve/carbo-load process before the event.

Base training is the body's building process. To improve strength, endurance and speed over the long term, you must lay a sound foundation for the body or you invite injury. I've found it valuable to cross train for most athletes, unless you want to be the "best in the west" and then it's a little different. In building the base, athletes often do intense but slow, and then longer and longer, workloads. This safely strengthens the tendons and ligaments along with the muscles. Joint sprains and muscular strains result when you try to build or push the body too soon, because your tissue hasn't yet strengthened to match the workload. Muscles strengthen much faster than ligaments, which take longer as well to heal when injured since they have very little direct blood flow (avascular).

Building the base in the cardiovascular sense also improves heart and lung efficiency in delivering oxygenated blood to the tissues. That takes getting the body to work harder each time, progressively building. This teaches muscles to function and to burn fuel more efficiently. (See ATP)

Peaking

Runners, triathletes, cyclists, swimmers, boxers, and other athletes who compete in sports that require both strength and endurance use peaking. To peak, you devise a system to intensify your workouts to eventually simulate the event in which you want to compete in. As the event or race approaches, you decrease the volume of your training. During peaking, you decrease the amount of your workload or base endurance and increase its intensity or speed runs. In other words, a runner runs fewer miles but faster. A weightlifter lifts heavier weights but does fewer reps. A swimmer swims 20 or 25 miles a week instead of 50, but swims them faster. (The law of specificity dictates that you can't train at 7-minute miles to run a sub 4-minute mile race.)

Shortly before the time when you need to be at your best for a competition, you should begin a peaking/intensifying training and reduce its duration. How much or when to peak depends on the type of event. If it's a ten-kilometer race, many peak within a very short time, like one or two weeks. I know athletes that are always in peak condition; some of whom compete as often as once a month. However, they are a rare group, and in general they do shorter events. It's possible for some athletes to remain at their peak level for an extended time provided that they don't do very long events like marathons or the Iron Man. Many of the athletes I worked with were constantly peaking because they competed regularly in 10-Ks or short races. The problem I witnessed with this is that they seldom rested enough and they had aches and pains all the time. They did deal with it, many got massages, yet during this time the massage they get becomes just as important.

Peaking is a technique by which an athlete can arrange to be at his top performance level. Most athletes competing in the Olympics only peak once every four years. In the old days, it was thought that you could not peak more than two or three times a year.

Four to six weeks is usually the longest period that you can stay in peak condition if you want to compete at the highest levels. There are many weekend warriors who forget that the body needs to recover from competition, and they suffer the nagging, little, micro muscle tear syndrome. You have to listen to the body or you will fall prey to aches and pains even if you take care and eat right, get massages, stretch and otherwise do all the right things. Too many competitive athletes I have known over train. Recovery then takes longer, and injury is always near. "Listen to your body."

Peaking Too Early or Too Late

Premature peaking occurs when you are not being coached or you start your intensity workouts or speed drills too soon before the event. If you try to do more speed work to intensify and extend your peak, you will actually experience more fatigue or succumb to the overtraining syndrome. You will start to slow down, weaken and lose the edge you've gained. For example, imagine a weightlifter going for his all-time high of 450 pounds. He may steadily improve from 375 to 400, 425, and 435, and then suddenly he drops to 420. In this scenario, he has already peaked and now has to go back to building the base again. If he insists on peaking and working towards the higher weight, his performance will deteriorate.

It also happens in reverse in that you may start your intense workouts too late and peak too late for your event. This happens to some athletes in competition. It's too bad that many athletes I knew back in the '80s didn't even know about peaking. What I find astounding is that many athletes today in 2004 still don't understand peaking.

5) Reversibility

Even if you have worked out most of your life to stay in shape, you probably have found that you can't lay off for more than a week or ten days before all that you have worked for is gone. I mean dog-gone! Most of us trainers and many doctors don't fully understand why reversibility occurs so quickly, even among world-class athletes.

Their strength may remain for quite a long time, at least until muscles actually start to shrink, and believe me, even that happens especially after age 40. Athletes don't lose their strength or speed as quickly as their aerobic ability to sustain effort.

The factor that we see most readily is aerobic loss (a drop in the body's ability to use oxygen). In swimming, middle distance and long distance running -- these are the sports that burn large amounts of oxygen and noticeably lose fitness first. The muscle actually loses its ability to use and burn oxygen, as well as the heart and lungs to move the blood.

Reversibility sets in at a slower pace in strength for weightlifters, down hill skiers, and sprinters. To perform their events, these athletes don't need large amounts of steady oxygen and blood flow into the tissues. They will breathe much harder though as they get increasingly out of shape. They may run just as fast and lift weights that are just as heavy, but they will not be able to perform as many repetitions.

Besides a drop in ability and performance, another clue that you are experiencing reversibility is when you get out of breath easily, and when your muscles start to feel weak after prolonged use. Some people breathe hard just walking up a flight of stairs. Since muscles need oxygen at different levels for different uses, that activity of walking the stairs would demonstrate that the person is out of shape. The same is said when you get sore from a workout. This is the lactic acid response -- your ability to cleanse the body of lactic acid, a byproduct of burning oxygen, demonstrated by increased soreness. Of course, some soreness is common when you are building muscle and getting in shape. In fact, depending on your sport, you may have a constant amount of soreness for the duration of said sport (crazy, I know). As we said earlier, some athletes live with almost constant pain. However, this fact does not mean it's right or that it should be there.

Sports have become very specific because during the off season, the athletes continue to work on conditioning, flexibility and strength building at some level. They don't work on technique as much in most sports. In swimming, tennis or other more coordination-demanding sports, technique is continually used in the training program throughout the year. You can lose technique, too. All neurological coordination is subject to reversibility.

Because of reversibility, it takes far less time to get out of shape than it does to get in shape. Depending on your genetic body type and age, most people aiming for a good level of fitness can get in shape within a couple of months, depending on what their intentions are. To prepare for a marathon at age 40 can take up to four or five months. Reversibility can set in as fast as in a week or two, no matter what your fitness level.

Strength Plus Flexibility Equals Speed

This is one of the equations I have come up with that I apply to athletes. To increase strength you have to increase resistance as well as flexibility to the same motion that you will be making in competition. I would use the cat as an example: it's a small, thin animal that pound for pound is very strong. Even though their muscles are not big, cats are fast, very flexible, and can jump higher and run faster than most animals.

Likewise, by giving more freedom of movement to the human body's mechanical structure, it will perform at its highest level. With yoga and stretching in addition to flexibility, we also experience a sense of relief and a clearer mental state of being. Flexibility training will help not only athletes but also executives and ordinary people as well. We can all live better with increased wellness. It can not only reduce mental and physical stress but also reduce emotional stress. A muscle can move you and contract much faster if it is flexible and relaxed.

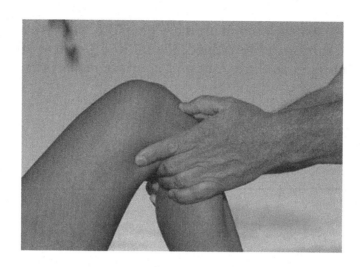

CHAPTER FIVE
STRUCTURAL BALANCE

To be structurally balanced means to be in harmony with a very strong force: gravity. If you're out of alignment, you're fighting gravity and from that will come tension, pain, and body aches. The skeletal system is designed to hold up the body and the muscles to move it. With improper posture or injuries we lose that function and create stress within the whole framework.

The pelvis is the foundation for the spine and the attachment to the legs. Any rotations, tilts, or deviations of structure here cause the muscles to work against each other and compensate throughout the whole body. The spine is also designed for strength and movement. Its natural curves disperse the downward pressure of gravity and are necessary for leverage and shock absorption. Like an effective shock absorber, the spine must also give, and be well lubricated.

Almost everyone has experienced some tension or pain in the neck at some point in life. One of the culprits is unhealthy postural habits. Looking down while reading, writing, or doing any hand-held activity invites gravity to pull on the head, which weighs more than the muscles holding it up. With long hours at a desk job, lots of tension builds in this area. It's no wonder that muscle tension in the neck, shoulders, and arms is so common.

According to some medical experts, up to 45% of adults over 40 years of age have potential frozen shoulder syndrome, or tight shoulders and neck. In a slouching posture, the misaligned shoulder comes out of its proper working relationship with the back and head. When the neck is tight and blocked it can affect the entire body, including the brain, often causing tension headaches or loss of concentration.

The muscles and bones of the body conform to your posture. If you are in any way misaligned, they stretch and contract to positions that are not balanced. Slouching shoulders, bent back, or a protruding neck can cause an imbalance in the body, all the downsides to poor posture. It gets to the point where it's impossible to just stop slouching, because the body has become skeletally skewed. We need to become aware of our posture in sitting, standing, sleeping, and walking to achieve good body balance. Knowing that the body has formed this way and acknowledging that most bodies have had injuries of some kind presents a dilemma. We can't just change it by suddenly forcing ourselves into correct posture. Muscles must stay contracted to put us back into correct posture, and we can't keep that up indefinitely. Gravity is constant, and if we fight it, invariably we lose. We need to be in harmony with gravity or suffer the consequences of tension, pain, and poor mechanical functioning.

Any postural imbalance in one part of the body causes something somewhere else to compensate. The gravity line is very specific: If something in the body moves forward, something else must move back. If the body is out of balance, muscles are pulling inconsistently and asymmetrically; some are overworking, others under working. Muscle spasms can increase tension in the joints and from there the spine, increasing the pressure on the discs. The disc pressing on a nerve is the cause of most back and neck pain. These are responsible for causing pain and loss of energy. Due to this constant tug-of-war, muscles fatigue more quickly than they should, wasting a tremendous amount of energy. Also, during rest, muscle tension can create anxiety that can begin to undermine the overall function of the human body. Structure governs function. Loss of sleep, impaired digestion, and shallow breathing can lead to more serious problems over years of prolonged tension.

With proper spinal and pelvic alignment, the body functions at high efficiency. When the alignment is healthy, we have more available strength, freer movement, increased endurance, and (best of all) much less stress on the spine and joints.

Rest

Structure governs function; the organs cannot fully do their job in an over-stressed, misaligned body. Athletes put their bodies through constant stress from training and bodybuilding. That's why rest becomes a very important factor in training, especially for competition. Many people in competition over train, blindly following the idea of "no pain, no gain." More and more research proves this claim to be false.

We need to look more closely at pain on the level of training in individual circumstances. We are all individuals, unique not only physically, mentally and chemically but emotionally as well. We're all so different; hard training for one person is easy for another. It's difficult even to compare two people of similar age, physical condition, and temperament.

Correcting Imbalances

The key to intelligent training and fitness is to work on balance. Consult with a professional to develop the basic structure for your workouts, and then follow those recommendations to the letter. Your body will be in better shape and it's likely that your stress levels will decrease. Body balance in sports is very important for performance and injury prevention (see sports massage section).

The most important corrective factor in total body alignment is the strengthening of weaknesses. Body therapy like chiropractic care, Kinesiology, structural integration, and deep tissue massage is very helpful when applied properly, however, this is only part of the equation.

Shortened muscles must be massaged and lengthened with exercise and conscientious stretching. Proper stretching and deep muscle work can be very beneficial for an athlete or any person in training for that matter. Changing the body into its proper structure takes tremendous knowledge, follow through, and dedication. Strengthening the weak muscles is the other part of the equation, and always making sure to balance the antagonist muscles as well.

General health as well as top performances comes from several factors besides training, eating right, and resting adequately. From the muscle standpoint, if you have an imbalance in the main muscles of the pelvis or legs (which many runners have) you can tap into only a fraction of your power because of your muscular imbalance. They don't work quite right, sometimes causing a shortened gait, inflexibility, and diminished strength, not to mention the muscular tug-of-war that causes fatigue and sabotages the body's mechanical efficiency.

You may think weightlifting is the only solution -- not so. If you build up muscles without the proper balancing, you just exaggerate both your strengths and your imbalances. Muscles have immediate communication with the brain. If they are very stressed or in danger of injury, the brain throws a circuit breaker to shut them down.

Here's where the problem is: Through a muscle evaluation (Kinesiology) you can determine which muscles are working and which ones are not. It's like tuning a car. If it's not working right, running it harder or just letting it rest will not correct the problem. If a wheel is out of balance, giving the car a tune-up will help it run better, but you still haven't addressed the imbalance. Each branch of body therapy (and of medicine) works on a specific situation.

One of Dr. Weil's wisest sayings is:

> *"Do not seek help from a conventional doctor for a condition that conventional medicine cannot treat, and do not rely on an alternative provider for a condition that conventional medicine can manage well."*

To get the most out of your body and your training consult with sports medicine and health centers that specialize in sports therapy techniques such as massage, Kinesiology, or fitness training. Don't underestimate the importance of having a proper analysis of muscles in your body, so you can identify your needs. This will address the structural balance of the body. Of course, it's all connected. Early on in my career as a massage therapist, I learned how closely the brain is involved in healing the body; it's a oneness.

Chemical, Structural, Electrical

Acupuncture works with the electrical system of the body. Chiropractic works on the structural part of the body. Herbs and nutrition work on the chemical part of the body. Acupuncture, acupressure and trigger points all work on the electrical part of the body. Some other forms of massage like Tragger, Feldenkrais, and polarity work on the electrical system as well.

Sports massage however is primarily concerned with structure and chemistry. Again, we'll simplify the point by comparing the body to a car. Tuning up the car makes it run better, but if the wheel (structure) is out of alignment it will drive terribly. If you put the wrong gas in the car (chemistry) it may not run at all! So if you work on the problems with the right tools, you can expect better results. You could get any massage and it will probably feel good. The results that you get depend on what you want.

They all have their place even within the body and structural part with different systems, like massage, yoga (this crosses over to mind work), physical therapy, etc.

HOLISTIC APPROACH

The holistic approach incorporates body (structure), mind (relaxation, mental imagery), proper breathing techniques (as in yoga), and high performance attitudes (spirit) while training. Nutrition establishes your chemical balance. You can help balance the body by developing a personal nutritional program that you can live with by eating the proper foods, avoiding the not-so-good foods, and having the correct proportions of vitamins and power foods. (See nutrition chapter.)

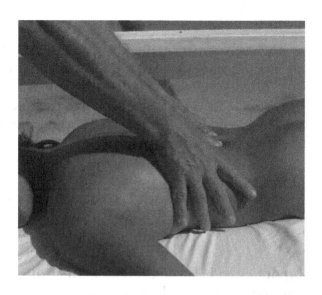

CHAPTER SIX
Massage Therapy

Massage has been known for thousands of years to promote wellness. Every culture in the world has some ancient form of massage; they are all wonderful for the body. How and what it can do for you depends on the type of massage therapy specifically administered to you, as well as what your beliefs are about it and the needs you have at the time. The most common is a form of Swedish massage, but as techniques and awareness grow, the technique and style will depend on the therapist doing the work.

Well-trained massage therapists can use their knowledge and hands to create a well-balanced body as well as a relaxed state of mind for their clients. Massage can be an important adjunct for any rehabilitation or sports therapy. The key is in the training and orientation, as well as the deeper understanding that we can relieve symptoms, we can be great healers. However, if we do not teach and encourage others to live their own healing, the body will constantly out-picture disease or pain, if there is such a thing. (Cotting) I believe our bodies always choose to serve us. Let's go on.

The benefits of massage are like anything else in fitness -- you have to do it regularly to get the most benefit, just like with eating, jogging and other sports. If you get a massage once a year or less, you are so tight that it takes a few hours just to loosen you up. One hour just doesn't make it; it may take longer, along with a good soak in a hot tub.

The origins of therapeutic or medical massage started with the common instinctual need to hold and rub a hurting back or pain anywhere. We humans like to touch and be touched, and we use it therapeutically as well as for showing affection. It can be very reassuring to be touched with care and knowledge, it's part of human nature, well, for most of us. There is enough research to not need to get on that wagon.

All cultures in the world have some sort of massage system and they go back thousands of years. Well, maybe more. How old are we humans? I imagine massage goes back as far as we have had bodies and gravity to work with. Now, with modern medicine we holistic practitioners use massage as an adjunct to health and fitness as well as physical therapy.

The father of modern medicine, Hippocrates, taught that massage was very important for any health program. He was one of the first in Western times to employ it according to some books. The Romans, the Greeks, the Chinese, the Hawaiians, and the Egyptians all did some form of massage. Did I leave out the Thais, the Olemcas, the... well, you get the picture.

In the last thirty years we have had a renaissance of health and wellness. This whole generation is very much going to change the habits of our fathers with the use of massages as well and with total fitness programs. We are in a spiritual renewal as well, and much of what we know as science is crossing over to spiritual. Since the *Tao of Physics* by Cappra we have seen many.

In ancient times, philosophers such as Permideus, Aristotle, and Socrates closely observed Nature trying to understand her laws and how the universe works. More recently, in the last century scientists like Newton, Planck, and Einstein, through their studies of physics continued to attempt to understand the nature of the universe and its laws. Some say that these same laws apply to the nature of human consciousness, that both the physics of our universe and the workings of our consciousness must obey the same laws, and many say these two are actually one and the same. Singularity right!

When Einstein first talked about the universe not having fixed laws, and thereby taking Newtonian physics to a new level, the scientists of the time asked that if the universe is moving, expanding and not fixed, how could we know anything. If it's always moving and expanding, there must be one thing that is a fixed point for us to know or study it.

Einstein responded with one of the most powerful statements of his career: "To know the universe you must pick a fixed point, and that is you! Once you do, you can understand the universe in relation to that fixed point. Then, getting together with another person or another point of view, sharing your information, you now know the universe from two points of view, and so on."

Oh my, that means, in a sense, we have to get together to know everything -- kind of a get-along-with-each-other philosophy. I like it. Working for peace was one way Einstein directly applied his beliefs. Many people say that he was not a religious person; however, I'm not sure what religion they were referring to.

For those of us non-scientists, this means that we can only know the universe or life from our individual point of view. Of course, the catch to this is that you must know WHO YOU ARE and that may sound redundant. You may say "of course I know who I am!" But knowing who you are also involves knowing clearly what you want from life, without any doubts. Any un-clarity surrounding these two main principles translates to the universe as un-clarity, and so then you don't truly understand either the universe around you or your life.

What we think is what we are, what we receive from life, and from the universe around us. In other words, it's all our creation. Our beliefs create our reality; our reality creates what we perceive; what we perceive creates the world around us, including our body, which we then "embody" into our selves. It is an eternal loop, and we are the center of our universe. Without us at the center there is nothing. THE UNIVERSE, LIKE LIFE, IS WHAT WE MAKE IT!

There is "a new kid on the block" and I have had the pleasure to take a couple of workshops with him. I've recently completed reading his new paper entitle "A Scaling Law for Organized Matter in the Universe and a New View of Unification." This young man, with Elizabeth Rauscher, has written the law that Einstein spent the last twenty years of his life trying to work out, "The Unified Field Theory."

There is so much within this information that applies to science, astronomy, and physics, but more importantly, to how we live our lives. This is the most important aspect of all this new information. Well, it is for me, and I think it is just as much so for everyone who questions the usefulness of all this knowledge and physics, and wonders "what does this all mean to me in my every day life."

What it means, of course, is that we are each ultimately responsible for our own life and the universe around us. Some people agree and then say in the same sentence "yes, I'm responsible for everything in my life, well, everything that is, except the time that tourist ran into my car." Well, it doesn't quite work that way -- it's all or nothing.

It presents us with a host of questions: If I create my entire universe, then do I create my own pain and my own illness? And what about disease: Is there being in-balance in the universe, and can I ever be out of balance? Is there death? What about a paradox -- can there be paradoxes in the universe?

Are you afraid of what you really feel? Do you concern yourself with what other people think of you? Are you running in a race that seems to have no end? What do you want to do with the rest of your life? Well, excuse me, I don't mean to get so personal, but I truly want to see all of us living the truth of ourselves whatever that is. If we want to fight the system or foolhardily support the system, either one keeps us in struggle. You just have to be yourself whatever that is for YOU! That's all that matters: You. Now, when you can truly be YOU, you can be with all the rest of us. Why be someone else you say? Well, there's our parents YOU, our society YOU, and your own limitations of you. Because truly only YOU can limit YOU. That does not make us selfish, as you can only be conscious from your point of view.

The universe is what we create, it did not create us! Well, actually it's simultaneous like Einstein said. We constantly create our universe as we go, and it creates us. A black hole is not devoid of light. It is the focus point of all light and all what we call dark, but it does not make it duality, it is actually a singularity. That is what all the physics is showing these days (Einstein, Nassim, Haramein).

The point is all these ideas relate directly to healing. We need to understand what the body is saying with the pain, because usually if we don't listen at one point, it gets louder and louder. So, get a nice relaxing massage; it's better for you.

Well, back to massage:

So, to just give each system its due, we will explain some of the basics that make up the different massage systems we employ.

Swedish Massage

A Swedish fencing master originally developed Swedish massage in the late eighteenth century. This was one of the few systems with the application of therapeutic massage in the West. It was based on some of the European folk massage, oriental techniques from the Middle East, and some of the knowledge of anatomy and physiology.

The strokes and manipulations of Swedish massage are each conceived as having a specific therapeutic effect. One of the primary goals of Swedish massage is to improve circulation of the venous blood from the extremities, as well as flushing the tissues and increasing lymph movement towards the heart. Swedish massage assists in sports or tension recovery by assisting the elimination of toxins like lactic acid, uric acid, and other metabolic wastes. It can also increase circulation without increasing heart rate like when working out. It's known to reduce high blood pressure and hypertension. It stretches and mobilizes the muscles and tendons keeping them supple and soft. By stimulating the blood flow it stimulates the skin and soothes the nervous system as well. It's one of the best systems to reduce stress, both emotional and physical.

It has some variations, but usually the strokes are deep and firm following the muscles towards the heart, with softer lighter strokes away from the heart to the extremities. Circles are done around tendons and joints to assist in increased circulation and movement in the joints.

Shiatsu

Shiatsu is based on the Chinese theory of acupuncture meridians and points. Its main purpose is to assist in the circulation of the subtle energy, or Chi. We use meridians running through and over the body, which ultimately connect with the nervous system, internal organs, and thus our entire electrical body. Through these points the therapist can effectively stimulate this energy. This massage can be deep, and because the pressure on these points usually has localized pain, you may experience some discomfort. This is like trigger point therapy, not very pleasant while being done, but great feeling after they stop. These points can be sore and by pressing them we create an escape valve effect and much of the pain and pressure is relieved this way. The key is to stay within the comfort zone. We don't think heavy pain will cure pain. However, deep seated problems in the body require some deep tissue work. Shiatsu also has some stretches, certain movements like rubbing, hacking, cupping, and other common massage techniques. It is a somewhat subtler form of energy work with the etheric Chi, prana or manna, rather than more of the gross structural work of the body like bones, joints, muscles, etc.

It's also good for stress reduction, relaxation, and a general improvement of well-being. Unlike Swedish massage, but like Lomi-Lomi, Shiatsu requires the client's participation with the therapist in coordinating the breath with the manipulations. It is a quiet and nice meditational type form of massage having very different results. Acupressure and reflexology work very similarly. They apply pressure on specific points for specific results, connecting through the nervous system.

Medical Massage

Although massage is not thought of in conjunction with western medicine, in Europe and in some clinics like ours, we have employed massage as a well tested practice for many years. In the U. S., we go to our doctors for most health problems. Some of us see chiropractors for our spines, or osteopaths who are well-versed in their arts or science. To me, they have to be balanced; we can all enhance our health and well-being much better by working together. After all, I am not all things to all people. It's the beauty in diversity that is the beauty in life. Massage can play as important a part as any of the other therapies and ways we live our life.

Medical massage can be used in rehabilitation with most simple injuries as well as the more intense ones like car accidents or surgery. It can prevent as well as reduce inflammation in strains or sprains with athletes. Even for the common sciatica or lumbago, which by the way are misleading terms, it helps by reducing muscle tension as well as releasing secondary holding patterns due to stress. It can also work to increase circulation of varicose ulcers, to stimulate normal bowel movements, and much more. The knowledge and the skills of the therapist determine the positive changes in many structural ailments that in the past may have had indications for not giving massage. Now the trained therapist is well informed as to contraindications.

Active and passive ROM (Range of Motion) exercise is the key to good structural freedom. The informed therapist may evaluate your range of motion and make recommendations for simple exercises to assist in balancing your body for better functional mechanics. The practice of yoga works to create a looser and relaxed body, and for various reasons massage and yoga go together well.

Lomi-Lomi

The history of Hawaiian Lomi-Lomi is very ancient, and there are also many styles. It has some very specific moves that make it unique along with specific breathing and movement patterns. It's important to understand the amount of energy and spiritualism that is part of this practice.

An essence of spirituality was what the ancient Hawaiians put into all that they did. There were many forms of healers including the herbalists, the fisherman, the hula kumu, astrologers, canoe builders, and the Lomi healer, to name a few.

These healers were called the "Kahuna." They were specialists in their particular fields and many times there knowledge was handed down generation upon generation. Many chants and rituals were part of their ceremonies.

Lomi-Lomi was a cherished style of body healing that still remains an important part of the Hawaiian culture today. I was fortunate to study with Auntie Margaret in Kelekekua and have also given her a few treatments over the years. She is now retired and just observes the classes.

We have applied this system by working with the circulatory and nervous systems. Through certain strokes and movements, the blood flow is increased, improving circulation and nourishing the muscle and tissues. The body metabolism is enhanced as muscle spasms decrease and toxins are flushed out.

As therapists, we approach our work with service with reverence. We have dedicated our lives to doing our forms of body therapies, hoping to increase the quality of life for all our patients and clients.

Sports Massage

This is one of my most favorite, all-around systems. Sports massage is primarily concerned with injury prevention, in my humble opinion. However, most often we do use it in the treatment of pain, chronic injuries, and over use syndrome, or in rehabilitation after acute injuries. The fact that it's called sports massage leads many people to think it's just for athletes. This is just not true. Sports massage is especially good for athletes, but everybody can benefit from it. It differs from other massage forms in that some of the techniques differ slightly from Swedish massage as the standard. It is a combination of some Swedish techniques but also includes Compression Massage, Cross fiber Massage and Deep Transverse Friction (DTF).

Compression massage is applied rhythmically with the palms of the hands pressing on the muscle. The object is to get blood into the deeper tissues while staying within the patient's threshold of pain.

In cross fiber massage, which can be applied with oil, strokes are made at 90-degree angles across the muscle and tendon. It is more commonly done with oil used on the belly of the muscle or on tendons by sliding the fingers on the skin over the muscle. This has many beneficial effects on the tissue systems including the reduction of swelling, adhesions, micro-traumas, and the increase of lubrication and blood flow. It can also be done in a more intense way without oil using the fingertips or palms more spread out.

DTF

The most powerful technique in all massage is Deep Transverse Friction (DTF) started by Dr. James Cyriax, an English orthopedic surgeon. He was the biggest proponent of this method, employing it for the majority of his patients' minor injuries. It has to be very specifically applied for it to be beneficial and to not create more irritation. DTF is a great technique for tendons, adhesions, micro-tears and musculo-tendonous joints and connections. Even on trigger points in the right areas, it can aid the body in accelerating healing.

Transverse friction is one of the best techniques for chronically tight or sore spots. (Read Dr. James Cyriax's books.) DTF also helps to increase motion by breaking up adhesions and also improves circulation to tendons and ligaments.

You need to be cautious when using this technique: you can irritate an injury worse with too much DTF. Used properly it can get rid a knot in a muscle, a sore tendon, or even a hot trigger point or torn ligament. This is great because using these techniques allow the athlete to go beyond what may hurt or limit him down the road. Many ligaments are re-injured because of poor healing and scar tissue. DTF promotes a well-functioning body; it's a valuable tool. Like all therapy when properly used on athletes on a regular basis, the pre-event massage improves the peak performance with fewer injuries and shorter recuperation time. Often we may do DTF with ice every other day until there is improvement, and then start with the fingertips again.

We could write a whole book on DTF and some doctors have (Cyriax). Applying transverse friction to the tendons (origin and insertion) and progressively going deeper with each treatment, you can take so much stress away from a joint that it makes a huge difference in competition as well as in everyday life. I don't do DTF only on athletes -- heck, everybody needs it.

In general, sports massage or corrective bodywork sessions are done with three or four sets of compressions alternated with three or four sets of deep transverse friction (DTF).

We normally will take one muscle group at a time. I usually begin with the biggest muscles first and work my way to the smallest, from the belly of the muscle to the tendons, and from the tendons to the ligaments.

Injuries

The usual athletic injury, whether due to a direct blow, tear, or to over-stretching, results in the same pathological tissue damage. A muscle spasm is the first sign of injury, and if you push it further the signs intensify. Tissue death and blood seepage from vessels and capillaries create a hematoma from a blow or tear. This is a mass of tissue debris and blood with extra calcium and other chemicals that the body dumps into the system. It's shocked, and everything binds up to protect it.

Following the injury and shock comes the inflammatory response, which creates an enlargement of the original hematoma. It's the body's cast: white blood cells and nutrients are sent to the site, including extra calcium, to repair the damage. The problem is that it backfires by causing tissue death due to slowed blood flow and oxygen starvation. As soon as the initial trauma occurs, this cycle can be broken with the application of RICE, which stands for Rest, Ice, Compression, and Elevation. RICE is the preferred treatment plan for most injuries because it minimizes the damage from secondary effects and accelerates healing.

Pre-Event Massage

A pre-event massage is mainly used to improve an athlete's speed, power, and endurance. It can help them perform at the top of their ability. We've seen it over and over: an athlete that is balanced structurally is one who has learned to strengthen and stretch the right places. Obviously, a well-balanced, well-timed and properly built machine, which the human body is, runs better. Sports massage is used for injury-prevention in the athlete more than any other type of massage. This is because of the way it's designed and the ultimate results you are seeking. Structural balance is the key by reducing the trauma from training and allowing the athlete or the executive to train and work harder and still recover faster. Besides, recovery massage helps the athlete and executive to be at a peak, relaxed muscle level, and it also helps to enhance mental clarity.

The pre-event massage is usually not done very deep unless the client is really used to it, but even then, we don't do deep work other than with deep compressions before the race. We sometimes use a combination of effleurage, petrissage and direct pressure on tight areas, mostly tendons. We may even use a little Deep Transverse Friction (DTF), or Circular Friction, as a post-event treatment. You need to take care and take into consideration the amount of therapy the athlete has had, as well as his possible conditions. I have seen athletes get some very good deep massage and run badly afterwards. They were not used to it, and it diminished their performance.

The usual effects of the pre-event massage are enhanced circulation, loosened muscles, and improved cellular nutrition through the dilation of the capillaries by deep compression or massage.

Rehabilitation Work

Sports Massage is also valuable in rehabilitation work. Unfortunately, the majority of the problems we see in the clinic are injury related, generally resulting from contact sports or from over training. Often it's patients recovering from auto accidents that can benefit highly from DTF. When players push the envelope in competition during sports, trauma often results. Injuries are incurred when the body is forced beyond its established foundations. This causes many problems among runners and other intense athletes. (Refer to laws of training, building a base). With massage and icing we have assisted many injuries in recovering in half the usual time. We can only really assist nature, as well as teach the patient what they can do to live their fitness level or heal from an injury.

Post-Event Massage

Post-event sports massage is used primarily for recuperation from an event, race or an intense training session. I recommend that any athlete who is serious about training get a sports massage from a knowledgeable therapist at least once a week. You're investing a lot in your body, and just like a car it needs regular tune-ups. You'd still better be doing yoga or a whole lot of stretching.

The post-event massage will speed up the recovery after an all-out effort in training or a race, and will aid in removing the lactic acid, free radicals, and other toxins while promoting great relaxation. Most athletes are so charged up you've got to get them to come down off that race. Trigger points release tension and spasms can be stopped with compressions or with circular friction, another form of DTF. It also takes a lot of stress out of the nervous system. There is origin and insertion work in Kinesiology that helps muscle spasms (refer to that section).

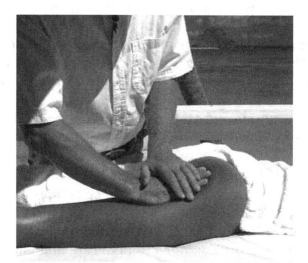

Techniques For Compression

The essence of compression work is deep, repetitive pressure to the belly of the muscle. This promotes circulation to the deep tissue and is more tolerable than using the fingers or DTF. Usually the therapist finds a knot and applies the technique to it for a few minutes. The compressions should be administered in a nice rhythm, always breathing with the patient and applying the pressure with the exhalation. Stay within tolerance: never go into pain. Remember, you can't fight pain with more pain.

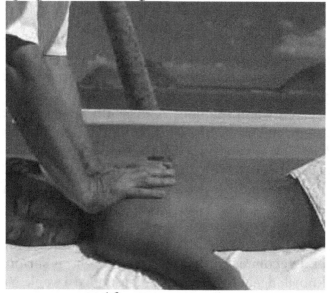

Wide, Deep Strokes

With wide, deep strokes (Swedish, lymphatic) we cleanse the body. We're aiding in its elimination of toxins, as well as in circulation and the movement of lymph and blood. This is what happens at the chemical level. A full body massage can take from 60 to 90 minutes to complete. This is sometimes tough to make time for these days when everyone gets so busy. Like I said, if you are a dedicated athlete or an intensely active person, massage is a necessity not a luxury as some people think. I used to do full hour massages, and sometimes an hour and a half. It all depends on the situation as well as what you are trying to achieve. In the different clinics I have worked in, the length of a massage varies from 15 minutes to an hour.

I go for more for frequency rather than intensity. While some of this massage work must be deep to be effective, you still have to stay within the person's pain tolerance. You can do deep tissue work without pain by slowly building up over the course of several sessions. I don't try to do the deep tissue work in the first session. You can go deep by slowly increasing the pressure as you work with someone. They didn't build that body in a day and you can't help them in one session to change it. It takes time, knowledge, and care to build a structurally aligned body. Massage can help, but it also includes proper training, good nutrition, yoga, and the right exercise program to structurally correct muscular imbalances.

Acute Conditions

Muscle spasms or cramps are acute conditions that can be stopped with deep compression (just grab hold of the cramp), or origin and insertion techniques (push muscle together from the origin and insertion) from Kinesiology. Spasms have way too many causes to list here, but usually in order of frequency it's from over use of the muscle as the most common reason, the lack of water, and the lack of electrolytes (minerals).

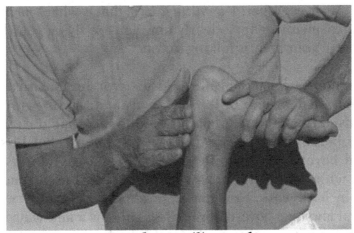

DTF on the Aquilies tendon.
Adhesions

Adhesions and other abnormalities in the belly or other soft tissue of the muscle will be addressed through friction (DTF) and direct pressure (Trigger Points, shiatsu or acupressure). For more detail on specific treatment, see sports injuries treatment.

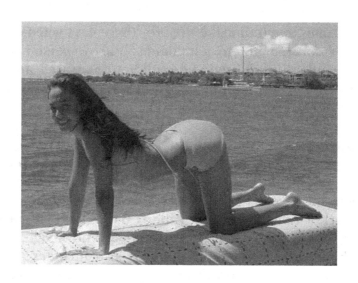

CHAPTER SEVEN
YOUR BACK

The back is the strongest part of our bodies and yet it is the source of one of the most common ailments of our civilization. It is built of strong bones, ligaments, and large muscle groups. Yet through bad posture, lack of muscle tone, improper lifting, and just plain ignorance, we constantly do our backs harm. Between 80 and 90% of all adults have had some sort of back or neck problem in their lives and will continue to have them until we change everything in our lives. What? Everything? Yes, that is what I mean; it's about all your life. The back is just out-picturing very clearly how you are living your life. Pain is intense, self struggle of some sort; your body is talking to you.

Everyone knows someone who has ruptured a disc, or has sciatica or some low-back syndrome. This is what we deal with by having a body and fighting gravity. It seems we are losing the battle, considering our aches, pains and the fact that gravity will kick our butts everyday. We suffer because the body is a moving structure that lifts, bends, runs, and sometimes is pushed beyond its capabilities. When we were hunters and gatherers, we worked in harmony with nature and gravity. Or we at least used time-tested methods to strengthen the body by hard work. Now that we are more "civilized," we've lost touch with nature and the natural laws that govern our bodies. There is a new way of thinking, too, that asks since we do create our own realities, what is this back pain saying?

We have grown out of shape and we struggle not only with nature but often with ourselves, and with other people as well, and we have become tight. Stress was born in the caveman times; we didn't invent it, we've just improved it. The "fight or flight" response remains evolutionarily embedded in us, no matter what. It is as ancient as our bodies. How we deal with this physically and mentally determines our health and the harmony we live in.
So, modern man has put the body to the test. We have increased the stakes in the game of life with modern business.

Who is in the driver's seat? In other words, who is in control or out of control in your life? Most of our stress, I hate to tell you, is "self-imposed." We make it all up as we go...

Executive Fitness

Now high-level executives have begun to realize that having the edge in business is just like an athlete having the edge in competition. At present there is a trend among executives who have the sense to use fitness and the right training for the body and mind. This epitomizes the competitive, high-powered world of modern business, the "type A's" with their competitiveness in sports as well. The winners understand it takes tremendous energy and concentration. The key is to know how much energy your body can produce when you train it as a whole. Add the mind training and you have the holistic approach to training. Then you can live your life as you truly desire.

"High tech, high touch" is a term I have used for close to 20 years. Our hereditary traits, our work environment, our physical activities, and sports injuries affect the way the body carries the stress of gravity. Also there are life's little moments, mental stress and emotional family neuroses -- need we go on? To make it short, all of these factors are part of the equation of what is going on with our bodies. You are the sum total of all your experiences, events, beliefs, and attitudes that you have lived with all your life or lives, if you get my drift. Consequently, our back is a reflection of all of that, which can make it complicated -- even we doc's have problems understanding the back.

By the time the pain is severe enough to see a doctor, there's not much most doctors can do. It takes five to ten years to deteriorate into that condition, so saying "Doc, fix my back" is like saying "Hey, correct my life of the last decade." No matter if you go to an orthopedic doctor, a chiropractor, or a therapist specializing in backs, it's going to take time and effort on your part to re-educate your body. It takes a big commitment to heal yourself naturally. Drugs and surgery should be the last resort, and most doctors now are conscientious about this.

Doctor Bernard Portner is a specialist in Physical Medicine and one of the best back doctors in the state of Hawaii. He was the former director of the Back and Neck Clinic at Straub Clinic in Honolulu and has had his own very successful practice for many years. Dr. Portner says:

> "Most back pain gets better responding to time and proper treatment. If treatments are going to be effective, a noticeable improvement should be seen within a few weeks. If no improvement is seen, question whether the treatment is worthwhile and seek alternative treatment. The trick is education. Learn to prevent further back problems with correct posture, proper lifting techniques, and correct exercises."

Exercise is the key in preventing back problems and in correcting and re-educating your body. "How long do I have to do these exercises?" is the question many of my clients ask. "Forever" is my answer. Health is an on-going state and constant exercise is required to maintain it just to counteract the daily stress the body is subjected to along with the mental state, since it is all really one. In order to get and keep your back in prime working condition, you must make the commitment. The right exercises will help correct your posture, keep your joints flexible, and strengthen the necessary muscles to maintain your back health.

Let's look at posture. You've heard since childhood to "sit and stand straight." But do you know why? Well, in actuality the bones must hold the body up with very little muscle action. When you slouch your muscles are pulled out of their normal working position. If it becomes a habit, they grow that way. The muscles can no longer work properly to keep the body in harmony with gravity. That improper posture causes stress. The resulting symptoms are aches, pains, and a constant tug-of-war in which tense muscles work against each other and lose their functionality.

Flexibility

To regain flexibility is the only answer. Without flexibility, the joints (including those of the neck, spine, hips or lower back) become more prone to ongoing stress. This is why we need stretching or yoga to keep the body limber. To reduce the stress, the body must be worked in opposition to the pull of gravity.

Once your skeleton becomes misaligned through habitually poor posture, and your muscles become accustomed to the resulting asymmetry, the cumulative effects of the muscular tug-of-war and of gravity take their toll. With certain movements "you can throw your back out" as we've been warned. But you don't just bend over and throw your back out; this is a situation that takes years to develop. A certain movement may create a muscle spasm or may pinch a nerve severely enough to hurt or temporarily paralyze you. However since the back is so strong a tissue, bone, cartilage and ligaments, it must be time and focused stress put on the ligaments and discs. This leads to most of us humans that sit all day at our jobs, we know that you increase the stress on the spine when you sit as the legs usually take up the shock of gravity. You exert 50 to 80% more weight on the discs when sitting.

The most common muscle spasms occur around a nerve and produce a weak or dull ache in the back or neck. Most often, the main culprit of all this pain is the disc, the soft tissue between the vertebrae. When a disc swells from too much pressure, or tears from a severe strain, it protrudes and presses on the nerves. This is the major problem. It can be corrected, but it takes time. Your body wasn't built in a day, and you have been alive, how long? The longer you've had the problem, the more you need therapy, strength and flexibility training, and nutritional guidance to correct the problem.

Strength

Strength is the final element necessary for a healthy back. If you've never exercised and your muscles have no tone, or if you do only certain exercises, you're probably out of muscular balance. The most common problem is weak abdominal muscles, which cause stress to be transferred to the lower back. A lot of people only use them in the morning to get out of bed. Exercise to increase abdominal strength is one of the most important components for a healthy back. The problem is that many abdominal exercises are commonly done incorrectly.

Another big problem is that some stretches or exercises can help some people, yet hurt others. The best way to build up your abdominal muscles is by first strengthening the deep stabilizer muscles in the pelvis (See section on the Laws of Training and building a base).

We have to build the ligaments, the deep muscles, and then the larger surface groups. For the abdominal muscles, proper crunches need to be done without pulling on the neck. Straight ahead (rectus), to the side (oblique), then modify from there. As you can see, even simple exercises can get complicated.

Building anything takes time and knowledge. To build any body, first it must be evaluated, and then it must be properly aligned. If your body is not balanced then you'll only magnify the imbalances, if the structure isn't corrected first. Your exercise must be consistent for the outcome to be good, so it helps to have a good program to follow. (See Training section.)

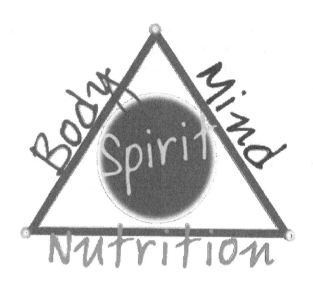

CHAPTER EIGHT
CHEMICAL/NUTRITIONAL

"It's what's eating you that counts." Dr Bruce Parker

Oxygen is the most important element in life. Carbon, hydrogen, nitrogen sulfur, and oxygen are the five elements of all life. These are the elements all things on this planet are made from. Oxygen is the most abundant, and when you think about it, it makes up 50% of the earth's atmosphere. It makes up about 40% of all vegetation, 85% of the seawater, and 45% of the soil. It makes up about 65% of the human body.

As we said, food and water are essential but without oxygen we cannot live for more than a few minutes. We need it for all our vital functions since 90% of our energy of life comes from oxygen. The cells need it to function and regenerate. We cannot metabolize our food without oxygen, nor eliminate toxins. Our brain needs over 75% of the oxygen we breathe.

It's oxygen that enriches the blood, which is carried to the whole body, down to each individual cell. Many health professionals feel that it's the lack of oxygen that creates disease. Not only do we have lack of energy, poor vitality, and a weak immune system with lack of oxygen but we are also seeing much more disease. The research shows that our planetary oxygen levels are dropping especially in the cities, and if we continue to cut down the rain forests, we will deplete the largest source of oxygen on the planet.

The ways we lose oxygen in the body are as follows:
Stress, mental as well as from toxic chemicals in our food, air pollution and other drugs. Oxygen is the primary protector of the body. The stress produces more adrenalin and other hormones that utilize more oxygen. It is thought to affect the immune system. I, however, think that Cotting is right: our spiritual, mindful body determines the health of our immune system. In other words, your attitude towards life drives the overall health or wellness that you live.

Physical stress or traumatic injuries reduce the body's ability to circulate oxygen to the cell tissue. Infections are other physical problems. Your body produces "free radical" forms of oxygen that help fight viruses, and other bacteria. The research shows that many infections and viruses cannot live in high oxygen, as they are anaerobic diseases.

Oxygen combines with most every other nutrient to sustain our life:
Hydrogen + Oxygen = water.
Carbon + Hydrogen + Nitrogen + Oxygen = Protein.
Carbon + Hydrogen + Oxygen = Carbohydrates.
These are the most basic elements of life -- oxygen, water, proteins, and carbohydrates.

If we don't provide these basic nutrients in the proper amounts, the body will suffer and not work at its highest level. Many scientists now know that lack of oxygen contributes to many diseases. Oxygen therapy is a new emerging science and we have seen many cures brought about by this treatment. (Always consult with a physician before undertaking any form of treatment).

We have used everything from bottled oxygen, ozone therapy, and hydrogen peroxide (H_2O_2), which is still very controversial as it can imbalance your PH level and create more free radicals. The safest forms of oxygen therapy that are thousands of years old are "Pranayam," or deep breathing exercises.

The next most important nutrient we put in our bodies is water. Pure tap water is now almost impossible to find in most cities. Even here in beautiful Hawaii most people drink purified or filtered water, and sadly, much of the bottled water available today is of questionable quality.

Since our bodies are 75% to 85% water, it's imperative to avoid polluted or chlorinated water. By adding chlorine to water we are superficially attempting to purify it. While this might destroy some bacteria, chlorine alone won't remove the toxic chemicals that end up in our water source. Besides, chlorine has been linked with heart disease, and who knows how long-term ingestion may affect our health? Boiling water also kills some bacteria, but not all, so it makes more nutritional and economic sense to get a good water filter. This will help at least to get pure water into our systems. However, to get to the next level we need live water. The brain is about 90% water so it's essential to not only get pure water in the body but also live water to really nourish the body and brain. Using oxygen is a new form of making the water more vitalized as well as using other nutrients that you can add to water. (See the works of Victor Shalburger on live water.)

Fat

We're all aware of the fat revolution, and many of us have fought the Battle of the Bulge at some point. Even my 14 year old daughter reads food labels to see how much fat products contain. There are different categories of fat, and eating too much of the wrong kind of fat can compromise the immune system. For many years we thought that this led to heart disease as well, but there's some new research that links heart disease more to stress than to fat consumption. Most doctors are still telling us to cut down on both saturated fats (meats and milk) and polyunsaturated fats (oils).

Saturated Fats

Saturated fats are found in chicken, beef, lamb, pork, duck, and dairy products. It's a good idea to reduce these high fat foods and to modify your favorite recipes, especially if you eat them more than three times a month. Cut down on butter, margarine, vegetable shortening, and all products made with tropical oils and partially hydrogenated oils. A good guideline is to keep fat at about 15 to 20% of your diet.

Most people are making an effort to cut saturated fat out of their diets by reducing their intake of meat, removing the skin from chicken, eliminating whole milk and replacing it with 2% milk, etc. Read the labels and you may be amazed at the contents of the stuff you buy. Most packaged foods like cookies, breads and chips contain rancid oils, artificial colors, and preservatives.

Polyunsaturated and Hydrogenated Oils

Polyunsaturated oils, which are not that good for us either, include safflower, sunflower, corn, soy, peanut, and the dreaded cottonseed oil, which is downright toxic. These oils are unstable and many experts believe they react with oxygen and can damage DNA and cell membranes. Especially hazardous are the solid vegetable shortenings, and although butter is better than margarine, we should try to eliminate both of these from the diet. Hydrogenated oils are in lots of products as well; these are toxic to our cardiovascular system and should be eliminated.

Fatty Acids

When heated, unsaturated fatty acids form TFAs, or Trans-Fatty-Acids. Many doctors believe they cause damage to the body at the hormonal level and may jeopardize our natural healing processes.

Mono-Unsaturated Oils

I have always loved and preferred olive oil to all others, and it turns out that mono-unsaturated oils are the best for the body. They include virgin olive oil, canola, peanut, and avocado oils. These oils can help reduce the bad cholesterol in the body as well. Olive oil is healthiest and is best used raw, as in salad dressings or to drizzle over bread. Another good fat we can increase the consumption of is Omega-3 (fatty acid) by eating certain fish such as tuna, sardines, mackerel, herring, and salmon, salmon having the most. Some great vegetarian sources of Omega-3 that are gaining popularity these days are hemp or flax oil, or flax meal.

Carbohydrates

It seems that every few years a trendy new weight loss diet emerges. We've heard all these theories of weight loss: carbs are the enemy, eat more proteins, try the blood type diet, eat less, eat more ... it's confusing. I personally have tried many diets, not for losing weight but to experience them firsthand, for health and cleansing. Carbs are still a great source of clean-burning fuel in the body, especially for athletes. Carbs are only fattening if you're not burning enough calories because as we know, fat and carbohydrates burn clean, as long as you are eating more vegetables and not excessive carbs. It's only animal protein that does not burn clean; it actually creates toxic residue (see Protein Section below). Competing athletes often follow a strict dietary regimen, which involves monitoring carbohydrate intake to maximize their potential, a system known as carbo-starving and carbo-loading, is a fine tuning system that can help with competition.

Protein

We need protein to grow, maintain, and repair our tissues. These essential nutrients (amino acids) cannot be duplicated by the body, yet are found in other foods. In this country, very few people don't eat enough protein. Quite the contrary is true: most people in modern American society eat too much protein. Because of its complex molecules, protein is hard to digest. Even fat is a better source of energy than protein.

Animal Sources

Most people rely on animal products for protein such as meat, chicken, fish, and various dairy products. However, these don't provide an optimal energy source for the body primarily because animal protein is hard to digest. Worse, it creates a toxic residue in the form of nitrogen, which can irritate the immune system.

Eggs are a good source of protein, but shouldn't be over eaten. Get fertile, natural, free range eggs that are hormone free. Avoid raw eggs, since they carry a risk of salmonella quite often. If you like eggs, eat them once or twice a week, not daily. Balance is the key. Aim to get enough protein so that your body has enough for repair and growth, but not so much that the digestive system is overburdened by trying to eliminate the excess.

All this extra effort can deplete your body's available energy, leading to a build up of toxins, and contributing to a weaker system overall. Those heavy protein diets work to help people lose weight, but are not too healthy in the long run. Besides, protein is all about amino acids, and you can go straight to that source. The green drinks are the new salvation for getting the right nutrients into the body.

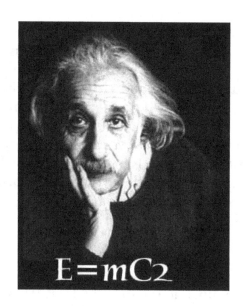

CHAPTER NINE
THE MIND

The Mind: What an Amazing Universe.

You are what you think. It's worth repeating. Scientists are now looking at the universe with very different eyes since Einstein. Let's look at "The Nature of your Universe."

In ancient times, philosophers such as Permideus, Aristotle, and Socrates closely observed Nature, trying to understand her laws and how the universe works. More recently, in the last century scientists like Newton, Planck, and Einstein, through their studies of physics, continued to attempt to understand the nature of the universe and its laws. Some say that these same laws apply to the nature of human consciousness, that both the physics of our universe and the workings of our consciousness must obey the same laws, and many say these two are actually one and the same. Singularity right!

When Einstein first talked about the universe not having fixed laws, and thereby taking Newtonian physics to a new level, the scientists of the time asked that if the universe is moving, expanding and not fixed, how could we know anything, there must be one thing that is a fixed point for us to know or study it.

Einstein responded with one of the most powerful statements of his career: "To know the universe you must pick a fixed point, and that is you! Once you do, you can understand the universe in relation to that fixed point. Then, getting together with another person or another point of view, sharing your information, you now know the universe from two points of view, and so on."

Oh my, that means, in a sense, we have to get together to know everything -- kind of a get-along-with-each-other philosophy. I like it. Working for peace was one way Einstein directly applied his beliefs. Many people say that he was not a religious person; however, I'm not sure what religion they were referring to.

For those of us non-scientists, this means that we can only know the universe or life from our individual point of view. Of course, the catch to this is that you must know WHO YOU ARE and that may sound redundant. You may say "Of course I know who I am!" But knowing who you are also involves knowing clearly what you want from life, without any doubts. Any un-clarity surrounding these two main principles translates to the universe as un-clarity, and so then you don't truly understand either the universe around you or your life.

What we think is what we are, what we receive from life and from the universe around us. In other words, it's all our creation. Our beliefs create our reality; our reality creates what we perceive; what we perceive creates the world around us, including our body, which we then "embody" into our selves. It is an eternal loop, and we are the center of our universe. Without us at the center there is nothing. THE UNIVERSE, LIKE LIFE, IS WHAT WE MAKE IT!

There is "a new kid on the block" Nassim Haramein and I have had the pleasure to take a couple of workshops with him. I've recently completed reading his new paper entitle "A Scaling Law for Organized Matter in the Universe and a New View of Unification." This young man, with Elizabeth Rauscher, has written the law that Einstein spent the last twenty years of his life trying to work out, "The Unified Field Theory."

There is so much within this information that applies to science, astronomy, and physics, but more importantly, to how we live our lives. This is the most important aspect of all this new information. Well, it is for me, and I think it is just as much so for everyone who questions the usefulness of all this knowledge and physics, and wonders "what does this all mean to me in my every day life"

What it means, of course, is that we are ultimately responsible for our own lives and the universe around us. Some people agree, and then say in the same sentence "Yes, I'm responsible for everything in my life, well, everything, that is, except the time that tourist ran into my car." Well, it doesn't quite work that way -it's all or nothing.

It presents us with a host of questions: If I create my entire universe, then do I create my own pain and my own illness? And what about disease: Is there being in-balance in the universe, and can I ever be out of balance? Is there death? What about a paradox -- can there be paradoxes in the universe?

Are you afraid of what you really feel? Do you concern yourself with what other people think of you? Are you running in a race that seems to have no end?
What do you want to do with the rest of your life? Well, excuse me, I don't mean to get so personal, but I truly want to see all of us living the truth of ourselves, whatever that is. If we want to fight the system or foolhardily support the system, either one keeps us in struggle. You just have to be yourself whatever that is for YOU! That's all that matters: You. Now, when you can truly be YOU, you can be with all the rest of us. Why be someone else, you say? Well, there's our parents' YOU, our society YOU, and your own limitations of YOU.

Because truly only YOU can limit YOU. That does not make us selfish, as you can only be conscious, think and act from your point of view.

The universe is what we create, it did not create us! Well, actually it's simultaneous like Einstein said. We constantly create our universe as we go, and it creates us. A black hole is not devoid of light. It is the focus point of all light and all what we call dark, but it does not make it duality, it is actually a singularity, which is what all the physics is showing these days (Einstein, Nassim, Haramein). Also called the event horizon by Nassim and others.

Let's start with the brain. It's the bio-computer of the body. It's the master organ that controls all the bodily functions of muscles, organs, glands, speech, systems, imagination, thoughts, etc. Well, it controls more than we are conscious of, that's for sure. Einstein actually said that imagination is more valuable at times than knowledge. He was the greatest theorist on human thought and the mind. He also said: "I'm not just showing you about mathematics and physics, I am showing you a new way of thinking." He was amazing; he is one of my heroes.

How can we more fully use this incredible computer for improving health, performance, and happiness? Where do we begin to learn how to use it? It takes training, practice, observation and understanding to be able to use the brain with control. Some people are capable of doing something perfectly on their first attempt while others need to try it a few hundred times before getting it right. It's critical to have someone who can guide you in using tools to get control of them yourself. Tools, time, teacher, thinking, trying, transcendence are all needed to begin harnessing the power of the mind.

The experts say we barely use 10% of our brains. I wouldn't be so sure about that or very proud of it either. Compared to other organs and systems of the body, the brain and mind remain largely unexplored. How many other functions does the brain perform or control that we are not aware of? What about treating the mind as a muscle? Athletes, businessmen, students and people of all types are looking into methods for training the mind.

The latest research shows that a loss of mental power doesn't have to come with aging. Now they say you can still build new neurons even into what we call old age, and that by exercising the mind like a muscle, we can strengthen it. In sports we do this by using imagery, relaxation, and mental clarity exercises.

There are other activities which strengthen the mind such as reading, doing crossword puzzles, learning a new language, listening to music and learning to play an instrument. Stop watching so much TV -- it's what I call mindless meditation, and mindless is what you get. As long as we work on both the body and mind, we will continue to have the best of both worlds.

We will now look into holistic training, which includes mind, body, nutrition, and spirit.

The first principles in mind training for athletic competition and excellence involve attitude and heart. Athletic endeavor is a way to tap into the deepest parts of the unknown mind and body. It's basically all attitude for the athlete, and that's also true for the rest of us. Your attitude determines your reality, thus simultaneously creating your experience.

This can be a great awakening experience, but unfortunately many of us get lost on the way to the park. We make winning more important so cooperation, friendship, peace of mind, and just plain fun often take the back seat. We often take ourselves way too seriously. We need to look at the attitude with which we approach sports as life. Do we love to compete for the sake of competition, or do we get upset and stressed if we lose? Are you pushing yourself to try and cause success, happiness or even health? Well, you can only live it if you can go out and cause it!

The most powerful mind space for athletic performance is fondly referred to as the "Zone." This refers to that deep state of mind/body where thoughts, trivial emotions, and problems don't exist. In technical terms it's called the "alpha state." Many people experience this zone or state, but the problem is that we often have little control over when or where we can experience it.

On the other hand, we want to be the best and so we train. In a joyous state of mind, we compete hard and when we lose, it's OK. If you set your goals inside and live them then you can make them happen. You don't drag the last competition around in your head; you get free of negative thoughts, focus, and imagine the perfect outcome. Visualization is one of the most widely used tools in sports. The coaches used to tell us "just imagine clearing the bar" or "close your eyes and see yourself making the basket." This was way back in the 50s and 60s. We hardly knew what it meant but we knew it worked. The research has been out forever; we just need to keep it simple and put it to use.

Our self-image in competition has a lot to do with our ability when the chips are down. It is in the heat of competition that our most powerful feelings and emotions surface. This is when the practice and mental training will matter most. We are affected at every level by past emotional occurrences that keep us from attaining self-mastery, starting with our most basic outlook. Knowing who you are is paramount.

Our outlook on the world, positive or negative, affects our personal power to create our own destiny. Ultimately, we are the masters of our own reality, and we must realize that we need to take responsibility for the outcome of all our actions. We create our results and must be willing to accept this fact to be able to master our minds to create other positive things. If you cannot change who you are, you have to change what you want!

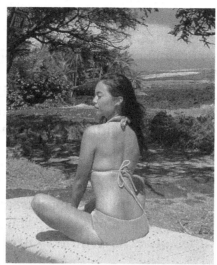

Concentration and Meditation

Concentration can be thought of as the Zen of mind training. In all athletic and life activities, the ability to concentrate is an important factor in building and preserving mental acuity. Learning to quiet the mind for pinpointed efficiency has been practiced for millennia by different cultures the world over. There are many paths to these great arts. I suggest meditation, tai chi and yoga, and offer a brief description of each.

Meditation

Athletes need to be able to completely relax and clear their minds for top performance. Why? Because any tension, not only in the muscles but also in thought, can cause constriction, hesitation, loss of coordination, and even pain! There are several meditative activities to quiet the mind. The difference between Zen and other forms of meditation is that Zen is the art of nothingness. Some teachers will direct you to focus your mind on the image of a black velvet picture and then to remove the frame. Others to just count your breaths by ten and just keep going. Thinking on one thing keeps your mind from wondering.

There also exist meditative traditions within the Christian, Jewish, Hindu and Tibetan faiths, which give you a word (or name) a prayer, a mantra (chant) or yantra (visual image) to focus on. Although these are still, non-moving techniques, they involve difficult respiratory, vocal or visual exercises to actively focus and prolong the concentration, and they should not be undertaken without proper guidance. We Westerners gravitate toward activities with some palpable, observable goal. We seem to prefer to strive towards something in order to facilitate that mind-body communication. So I recommend something that will be less boring to the majority something with movement in it

Tai Chi or Qi Gong

I highly recommend tai chi or Qi Gong, to everyone for the combination of power and softness it encourages. Its characteristic, slow movements teach total body balance and awareness. Most of all, it allows you to access the unseen and often untapped inner power called Qi or *chi*, or *manna*. Chi is the name given to the life force, or the energy present in all living things. In ancient times athletes were like warriors, saints or heroes, for they worked with a mighty force. This is what ultra performance is about--the "high" many athletes are addicted to. It's amazing how sometimes we forget our mind and follow the body around and do silly stuff because of the intensity of this energy. The women might say it's our testosterone, but I know female athletes who are even more intense than men. When you "hit the wall," these ancient disciplines allow you to call on this inner source of power, which lies beyond the physical and allows you to achieve great things. Qi Gong on the other had is similar in movement but focuses more on the internal healing of the movements.

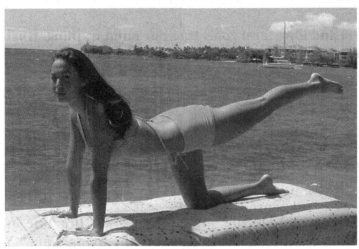
Yoga

I recommend yoga for flexibility and quieting the mind. Arguably, the most important aspect of yoga practice is the detailed direction of the breath. In the practice of physical poses (*asana*), the movement is always combined with the breath; this process keeps the body supple and the mind flexible. A body that is pliable, mobile, and strong will free the mind of physical worries and allow it to perform better. In a yoga class students are taught to accept their strengths and weaknesses, cultivating contentment (*santosha*). The resultant patience accessed through the integration of mind and body is a great tool for athletes. The other part of the equation, which is not necessarily religious, or anything so mysterious, is to find our own form of spiritual feeling. Once we achieve balance we can ignite the flame of the spirit. Whatever gets us in the "zone," is worth checking out. It's the ultimate sweet spot, for sports, love, and life.

It's stressful enough to just live on this planet in our complex inner worlds. For Type A athletes, who might tend to be obsessed, pushing the body and mind eventually leads to a breakdown at some point. We must train our wills, scientifically and spiritually.

We have the best of all worlds. We have the most up to date information available to us, plus all the ancient methods for ultimate balance. We have all the sports psychology, sports programs, doctors and research literature. We have marathons, triathlons, bike races, basketball ... you name it! We are going nuts with sports, executive fitness, sports training, mind training, spas, health foods. There is an explosion of information these days, so take advantage of it.

Great! What a blast we're having! It must be working, right? If not, it all boils down to this: If you can't apply the tools to achieve your results, either change the tools or change your mind. The key is you have a plan to get anywhere. As my friend Buckminster "Bucky" Fuller said, "It's 75% planning and 25% doing."

Summary for Mind Training

Most important, first figure out who you are, where you stand in the universe, and then decide how you want to play in the world and live your life to the fullest. Pull no punches!

(1) Set both short term and long-term goals for your mind training. (Include aspects of your life -- work, social, physical health and personal attitudes, for example).

(2) Clearly state your purpose, declare what you want, to live who you are, your purpose in life.

(3) List your priorities, the ways to enliven yourself and all those around you, for as you help others you find your way in the universe. Act as if you're already experiencing these changes. It may look like this:

> "My attitude has changed. I find myself living my life not by making more affirmations, more or positive statements, but really living them." You have to give anything you want in life away to have it.

> You can't program things into you, nor can you set goals outside yourself. You have to live it, not just hope for it or "think positive." There is no opposition in the universe; it's all part of the same "oneness." What you put your thoughts on is what you get and what the universe gives you more of -- what you want and more. That's the bonus.

> I still often meditate in the traditional sense or do relaxation exercises, but more importantly I like to live what I want at all times. If you have to think, or meditate on peace, you only create the struggle to have it; peace has to be a non-issue.

> While reclined, I focus on every part of my body, starting with my feet and working up to my head, relaxing in detail. "I want a new attitude toward competition. I want to be so centered with others that no one could take me out of my center. I never lose my temper in any situation. There is nothing I can't change."

> I'll take a course or do a workshop in yoga, martial arts, music, art or dance, and I will follow through, one thing at a time. Do whatever you may want to do, but first be you, and then what you do does not define or confine who you are. It can only expand you.

(4) Do your research. Find out what materials you need: tapes, books, a personal trainer or counseling. You can try out a couple of different programs before you commit, BUT DO COMMIT - HAVE FUN, IT'S SO MUCH FUN TO REALLY DIVE INTO A PROJECT!

(5) Ask yourself: What are the rewards for your perseverance and dedication? AND DON'T DO IT FOR THAT!!! LIVE YOUR LIFE FULLY!

The fifth step represents the most beautiful part of getting serious about anything in life. Once you get started, you'll see how your mind training overlaps into body training, offering an awakened, involved spirit as the prize. You'll find that nutrition is very important to mind training, (see nutrition section). Not only is it true that you are what you eat, but what you eat is what you think, too. Patience and perseverance in your mind training and in your physical training will add to the quality of your life, keeping you healthy in body, mind, and spirit. You can only live these things you cannot cause them. Understand that, for it is the most difficult part of this simple truth in life.

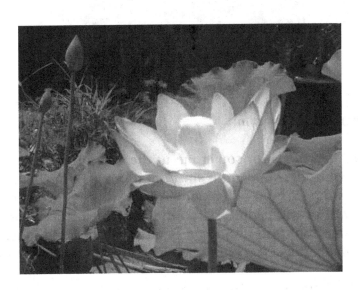

Enjoy life

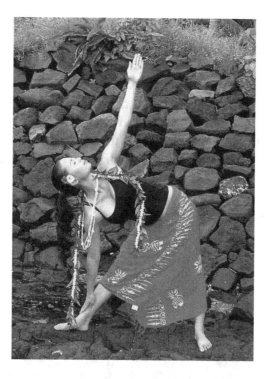

CHAPTER TEN
Aerobic Training

To start your aerobic training program:

Consider first setting your goals for sometime in the future; make sure they are realistic. Start easy, be kind to yourself. Many of us start out joining a gym and telling ourselves that now we will train every day! Six out of ten people going to gyms drop out in the first month. That's a staggering 60% of the people. The numbers are just as high for those that buy exercise equipment and don't use it. So you need several ingredients, not necessarily in order of importance, but because you want to be successful in your training.

1. Desire or motivation that is from who you are, not to get something.
2. Energy: This means you need to start thinking about eating better. No matter where you are with nutrition you can always improve (see nutrition for details). You need nutrients as well. Vitamins, power foods, high technology nutrition is available; you just need to make the effort. Without good fuel it's hard to get the energy to train.
3. Set your goals within yourself and make them realistic. Remember, there is no cause and effect so you can't cause health; you can only live it.
4. Make the time, create a loose schedule with alternatives, if need be.
5. Stick to it. Remember, consistency is more important than intensity.
6. Understand the basics of bio-mechanics, even for walking (posture, the muscles, the stretching, the meditation and imagery) to get the most from your efforts.
7. If you are in a family or a relationship, you need support and encouragement, not grief for leaving them alone so often. Get them to start with you (that's really tough sometimes). It's always easier if your partner is doing a similar program with you.

8. If you smoke, start making an effort to cut down, if that's really what you want to do. If not, it will not make a huge difference so much as your attitude towards it will. Use coltsfoot, an herb you can buy in health food stores and smoke it. It will cleanse your lungs, and help you to get off tobacco. You will find the desire will slowly fade away as you get healthier. We don't need to harp about it. JUST DO IT! QUIT.
9. If you eat more than a plate at a sitting, just start eating less, and limit snacks and fruit.
10. Maybe it's some of the food you eat. Cut down on fats, sugar, liquor, canned food, and packaged food full of hidden fats and sugars. I'm sure you already know the stuff that doesn't really help your body.
11. Eat more of the good stuff: fruits, vegetables, nuts, seeds, whole foods, grains, etc.
12. Drink more water, read more books, and have more fun in your life. Why not?

Of course there is more, but this would be a great start. Remember that when you work holistically you have a better chance at success. You will be working on several levels of health at the same time.

A few days you make it, then you miss one, and eventually another. I know, and I'm a professional trainer, it happens to me. Life is always changing, that's the beauty of it. That does not mean we give up; just go with the flow. Set some realistic goals, and know that you will miss some days. Make it up again, and don't beat yourself up about it.

The majority of people drop out of their health programs primarily because it is very hard to get motivated. There are a few myths about motivation for working out -- that knowledge will do it, or maybe we feel guilty because we are overweight -- but the key is if you don't have the energy none of that will matter. It's really about metabolism. Once you get older if you don't exercise, your own body will start to think you don't need the hormones and energy. Basically, it starts to shut down. When you do exercise, it's hard and your body feels like it's really stressed. It's not very pleasant, in fact, it hurts.

To really increase the energy level and have your body and brain work with you, you need to take the nutrients to get your body working again. The food you eat needs to be better quality with more servings of natural fruits and vegetables. If you are eating junky food there is no way your body will be able to have more energy. (See nutrition for more detail.)

You need to consider antioxidants, vitamins, and some form of growth hormone like DHEA. You can't take very much of this as it turns to testosterone and so you need to consult a doctor for medical advice. There is also IGF1 (Insulin-like growth factor), a precursor to human growth hormone. It's deer antler extract and very effective for improving your metabolism (see my web page for more information about this along with other nutrients). Most doctors don't recommend very high doses of either of these nutrients, so get professional advice. A small amount can do wonders for the human body. These nutrients increase metabolism, build muscle, and help the body to become anabolic (for building and repair). This is important: to not be catabolic (destructive down cycle) any longer. If you can use these health products, they are the best.

The research necessary to take the vitamin and nutrient business to its highest level is being done with these products. Your success in a fitness program is dependent on your nutrition program.

The minimum goal for an aerobic activity is five times a week for over thirty minutes each session, and even up to sixty minutes if you are only going to walk. Five times a week, not three times as we have heard. That doesn't mean it has to be all running or all walking. You can play tennis, golf, and walk briskly, or take a nice walk with the family. Families that train together, stay together. Play ball with the kids, for this to be effective and considered an aerobic activity, you need to do it over a half hour. By then you start to burn some fat. As you increase this ability to burn some fat your brain says "Hey! This person is active. Let's improve the metabolism."

As you exercise you also decrease your appetite so you eat less. This is when your body will start to create more hormones, endorphins, and pain-reducing substances called antefolins, which will help you to feel better. Remember, you have to get over the hump before you feel good from exercise. Then weight is not a big problem and you will slowly and naturally level off to your natural weight. This all helps to reduce your stress as well as helping you to feel more successful and some enhanced self-esteem. Balancing your body this way also helps reduce the risk of heart disease as well as diabetes. It helps you create more of HDL, which is the good cholesterol, and reduces the LDL & VLDL, the bad cholesterol.

A moderate exercise program always helps you sleep better. It enhances the digestion and the lymphatic systems (the cleanser of the body tissues). All this helps your body to work at the ultimate level. Remember, this is going to take time. Diets or any fast way will not last. We know now that when you diet or change anything too drastically your body goes into shock. Then the next time you eat, it holds on to it. You gain all the weight back.

So it's best to not focus on the weight. When your body is operating at its optimal level, you will be at your correct weight. It all depends on your body type, anyway. You could still be heavy and be incredibly fit and healthy. Isn't that the purpose of all this?

A sample schedule for the beginner fitness enthusiast:

Day One.

Take an easy twenty-minute walk at a nice brisk pace. (Walk ten minutes from your starting point and turn around.) Find a nice place to walk, away from lots of cars. If your neighborhood is good place well, great. If not, take the extra time to drive to a park, beach, pasture or the country. No sense huffing and puffing more carbon monoxide. (Living in Los Angeles is like smoking ten cigarettes every hour (Cherniscki)). You need to be able to keep up a conversation. If you are in oxygen debt you won't burn calories as well. Upon returning, spend about ten or fifteen minutes stretching.

Consistency is more important than intensity. If you don't do it regularly the brain thinks "well, this body doesn't need much energy so we can store all these extra calories in the thighs or butt." But if you start with some regular activity, just everyday stuff can contribute the message to the brain saying "hey we need more energy." The brain begins to think this body is active and needs to increase the metabolism. Every two hours do something for at least ten minutes. Then your brain will take you to a higher metabolic level. As you increase your exercise program you will have more byproducts called free radicals. This is more reason for us to work with nutrition as well, because you need to increase the antioxidants to keep the body healthy from the free radicals.

Day Two

Just stretch for ten to fifteen minutes. If you are near water, maybe swim for ten to fifteen minutes.

Day Three

Walk briskly for twenty-five minutes. Stretch for fifteen, or if you have it down, it could only take ten minutes to get a good stretch.

Day Four

Swim and stretch for at least twenty minutes and ten, respectively.

Day Five

You might miss one. . .

Day Six

Walk a good deal faster for twenty-five minutes. If you feel tight walking, stop after you break into a light sweat and stretch for ten minutes. Regarding the legs and gluteus muscles, see the chapter on the lower legs.

Day Seven

If you didn't miss one day, take an easy walk, swim or stretch, maybe do something with family or friends. If you got sore at all during the week, then rest and just stretch.

Continue this program until you can walk twenty-five minutes without losing your breath at all. This can take two weeks for most people and up to four weeks for others. If it takes you longer, stay with twenty-five minutes for two months, and then move into the next level. If within two weeks your body serves you well, you can proceed with the next level.

We will have an easy day and then a hard day for the rest of training. If you miss an easy day, don't worry about it.

Continue on the following day with a brisk walk for thirty minutes. Now we will start to burn some fat. From now on, you workouts should last about forty-five minutes. So give yourself an hour to work it into your daily routine.

As you get stronger, your easy days become more like your hard days when you first started. Walking can increase to five times per week within the first few months, depending on your body. You have to listen to it and pay attention. If you can get the advice from a certified personal trainer, please do. It never hurts to have more information. At this level it's not as critical as it will be when we start the strengthening program using weights or strengthening exercises.

Six to Eight Weeks

Most bodies will start to enjoy working out from here on out. After six or eight weeks, start your strength-training program. Once again, listen to your body. If you don't feel quite ready at six weeks, take eight. What's the rush? You have your whole life ahead of you. At this point is when I recommend the use of a certified personal trainer.

You can go in either of two directions with this addition to your program, with various levels of intensity depending on your body and your abilities. (See chapter on the laws of training).

If you are able and willing to run for your particular goals, you may now start to run. Start with easy jogging for twenty minutes every other day, and weight training every other day. Running at this time should be at least three days a week, the same for weight training. There is some evidence, however, that we could get by with two days of weight training (solid whole body sessions) and still do okay. Include one day of rest. The day you rest could be a very easy workout, either stretching or family fun.

For weight training we need to start just as easy. Many of us think that weight training will build large muscles. We see all these big bodybuilders, and although some of us admire the dedication it takes to build that kind of body, it is not necessarily true that weight training builds large muscles. It all depends on how you train, how much you train, and your age as well as the system of training. We know that by stressing any muscle naturally (exercises) or unnaturally (weights) we work with the law of irritation and adaptability to produce the result we want.

Basically, this means the body will adapt to irritation. Adapting can mean for size of muscle as well as for the functioning of the muscle. Adapting also can mean the heart and lungs adapting to more stress and improving the functioning of this system (aerobic conditioning). The irritation could be considered the stress exerted on the body (heart and lungs) by running or walking more and increasing time and duration. Then we consider strength in the muscles by more and more progressive exertion (making the body work progressively harder). This can be achieved by doing more and more pushups or other exercises. Using weight training for increasing strength, as well as burning more calories, we would have to build by lifting more times and more weight.

There is another way to use weight training to develop strength as well as endurance. This system works on the premise that using progressively more weight builds size and strength. Starting with more weight and then progressively reducing the weight with longer repetitions, we build endurance in the muscle instead of bulk.

It's widely known now that for older women weight or resistance training is beneficial to stave off osteoporosis.

Here is a sample schedule for the very beginning weight-training enthusiast:

Please note: This section is not to take the place of medical advice. I recommend that you speak to your doctor before undertaking any kind of exercise program, especially weight training. See a professional; it will be a good investment in your body. This schedule is suggested as an example of a very general training regimen and not intended to be used without help from a professional. It will give you an overview of the process of basic weight training. Each program needs to be specifically tailored for each individual in my opinion. (See the section on structural balance as well as other books by Molina.)

Begin by taking the time to become educated or be prepared to get professional help.

A Sample training program for maintenance. This is sometimes called:

Pyramiding down: This basically means reducing the weight as compared to pyramiding up, which is increasing the weight.

1. Get an analysis of your body. This means find out what muscles are out of balance and where your weaknesses are. This could save you time as well as a lot of pain down the road.
2. Always start with a warm up of some kind (Stationary bike, treadmill, aerobic class) to get your body sweating and warm.
3. Stretch before, if you have the chance or the time. If not, for sure stretch at the end.
4. Always start with the biggest muscle groups first and work your way down.
5. Start with about 75 to 80% of your maximum weight, something you can comfortably do for between 10 and 12 repetitions. Then progressively drop ten pounds each set. Do as many repetitions as you can in each set. As you drop the weight you increase the repetitions. This is less dangerous because as you become more and more exhausted, you have less and less weight on.
6. There is less chance of injury as you work with less weight. I have found that with this way, you will build endurance type of strength and not as much bulk. It helps trim your body as well as burn fat and create muscle.
7. For the upper body, start with the back muscles, the latissimus, trapezius, and shoulders and pectoralis group. Work towards the arms, biceps, and triceps. I prefer free weights to machines, as they tend to build all the support and peripheral supporting muscles. The machines do the supporting and thus you only exercise the major muscle groups. Machines are generally safer if you are working out alone and are okay for basic maintenance. Get a buddy or join a gym where you can get help. Eventually you will want to be using free weights.
8. For the lower body, start with the gluteus group (butt muscles), either in a squat machine or a squatting rack. Continue with the quadriceps, hamstrings and claves.

9. This workout can be done moderately in one full hour. It's very important not to rest between each set, keep moving from one to the other. If you sit there and talk, it could take hours. Remember, we have to build a base or we are inviting injury.

Go easy. Some personal trainers may take you over the edge, but you have nothing to prove, and if you can't walk the next day, it was too much.

Some soreness is bound to be there, you may not get it the next day as badly as the following day (forty-eight hours after). I recommend that you stretch for twenty minutes after weightlifting of any kind. Swimming or running the next day may be tough, so go easy. If you can't run after the weight training, it was too much. If the soreness lasts more than four or five days, you tore some muscle fibers. If that happens, RICE (See injuries) may help -- that's Rest, Ice, Compression and Elevation. This will be especially beneficial if you have specific painful sites. If you hurt all over, maybe the Jacuzzi will help or some massage. However, in my experience not much will help, including aspirin. It will just take some time to heal.

Day Two

Try to stretch ten to fifteen minutes after a warm up. If you are near water, maybe swim for ten or fifteen minutes if you are sore. If it's your day to run or walk and you can do your aerobic training, then go for it!

Day Three

If you have the time, it's great to warm up the body before weight training. Get on a bike for ten or fifteen hard minutes and break into a sweat. It's ideal to do a bit of stretching before, but far more important to stretch at the end of your session. Start your routine: Same as Day One.

Day Four

Swim or do your aerobic activity.

Day Five

You might miss one session, or you could be sore. Get a massage, which may be beneficial. However, if you are sore and you get a deep tissue massage, it will hurt. Soak in a hot tub and get a massage anyway, it's going to help regardless of the pain. I think this is where that "no pain no gain" expression comes in. Be careful, pain that does not go away after two or three weeks may need a medical doctor's attention.

At Four Weeks

Within four weeks, if your body serves you well, you can proceed with the next level.

Using weights for strengthening the body requires dedication. In our experience, consistency is more important than intensity. That means if you miss a day don't try to make it all up the next time. Four weeks may be the hump for many people. By this time your body is not getting as sore as it was during the first few days.

You have built a base and your body can continue to grow. You may start at more weight and by now you may also do a few more repetitions in each set. This could increase the time somewhat. However, if you increase the intensity you could still do it in an hour. You may be sweating and breathing hard. Once again, monitor your breathing; if you are gasping for breath you are working a bit too hard to get the most out of your workout. You can get an aerobic workout with weights in this method. Many people think weight training is only anaerobic (without oxygen) as compared to aerobic (with oxygen). It's this combination in the workout that gives you the endurance.

Eight Weeks

Now training becomes part of your routine. If you can stay with it this long you will be at the point where you start to see some of the benefits. You may be stronger, but at this time your body starts to look different. Your energy level will be better, and your weight may increase. WHAT ?! Yes, don't be surprised if your weight goes up just a bit. Or maybe you haven't lost any at all. Since muscle weighs more than fat, as you build muscle and lose fat you may gain some weight. Don't worry; it's at this point that the weight you are carrying looks a lot better than the old weight you were carrying around. Eventually you will lose excess weight if you were overweight before. The holistic approach will help you to find your ideal weight, which depends on your body type, family traits, eating habits, and on and on…keep training!

One word of caution, the weekend athlete seems to be one of the highest groups with small injuries. That company picnic softball game will cause pain not pleasure if you never workout take care with the once a year games.

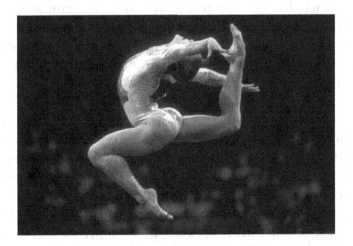

This beautiful body took a long time to build, yours should too.

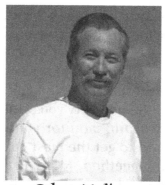
Othon Molina

CHAPTER ELEVEN
MY STORY

I have been a professional massage therapist, since 1970. For the first four years I had to supplement my income with odd jobs. I was fortunate to have been in the middle of the holistic health movement in the '60s, living in Los Angeles, the mecca of the mind/body revolution. Not only was our generation going through unprecedented mental, physical, spiritual, philosophical, and societal changes, we were in the middle of the Viet Nam War, sex, drugs, and rock 'n roll. Those were intense times. The profession of massage therapy has changed a lot since then.

Having been born in Mexico and then growing up in the States, I never quite fit in. I found myself starting out on my journey to self-awareness through sports. Sports were my meditation and what inspired me to greater heights. Running was my way of releasing stress, even though I didn't know I had any. When I was young, I would run in the desert of Mexico just for fun. Sometimes I would just cry like a baby when I was running, or have vivid dreams or visions. I didn't know then what it all meant and I didn't know what to do with it. It wasn't until later that I learned that my ancestors, the Tarahumara Indians of Mexico, were renowned for their running abilities. I also came to realize what the whole running revolution is about: getting "the natural high."

When I entered high school in Los Angeles, sports were my passion, but I found out that I was just mediocre as far as the measuring stick was concerned. Well, I did have some records and success as a runner, but I felt a little out of place, anyway. Looking at the two types of cultures gave me a kind of insight to human behavior. There were things I didn't understand such as the cultural, economic, and social differences among people. I had never felt that in Mexico; I thought all people were the same. Even though Mexican society is essentially a caste system, and socioeconomic differences are as big a problem there as in other parts of the world, I never noticed it much. There were attitudes and habits from both cultures that I didn't care for. So what I decided to do was get rid of the elements from both cultures that I didn't like and adopt the things that were good from both. I had the best of both worlds. Well, now I definitely didn't fit in. I was neither traditionally Mexican, nor typically American. (By the way, Mexicans are Americans, too.) We draw these lines between people, and I guess that is at times what separates us on this planet.

My interests went into studying psychology, but not in school, for I pursued a degree in architecture, something I really liked, too. But I started reading books and subscribed to *Physiology Today*, in high school for several years. I started delving into books on Zen Buddhism and religion, and studying authors like Alan Watts, Carl Jung, Kahil Gibran, Paramahansa Yogananda, and studying sacred texts like the Bhagavad-Gita, the Upanishads, the Bible and so on. Before I knew it, I was practicing Zen meditation and doing yoga.

Soon after getting into yoga, I was looking at a hamburger and thinking how gross this food was. That experience triggered my interest in nutrition. I read Ann Wigmore's *Diet for a Small Planet* and the *Muscleless Diet* among many others.

During those years we started experimenting with pot and other medicines like peyote and hallucinogenic mushrooms, which have been used for religious purposes by Native American cultures for centuries. To me, these substances were part of nature and needed to be used properly. I recognized that these healing remedies could potentially cure many people. Part of me is an Indian medicine man, part of me is a spiritual seeker, and yet another part of me is a scientist. I knew that most of my friends thought I was a bit odd anyway. In my opinion, most of my friends did drugs for totally the wrong reasons, such as escaping, dealing with stress, or for no reason at all, saying, "Let's get Fucked UP!" I used to say, "You're already fucked up, let's get awake." Weird, I know, but that's how I really felt.

My journey into healing lead me from sports to psychology, meditation, religion, yoga, and then to different healing systems like acupressure massage, polarity, reflexology, iridology, Kinesiology, exercise physiology, and all the "-ologies."

It became an obsession of study. By the time I moved to Guadalajara and transferred to the university there, it was 1969 and I had been studying healing for four years. I didn't know anything, but I thought I knew a lot. This was all reinforced that year when I met my first teacher, Evaristo Madero.

Evaristo Madero was a Yaqui Indian and a Curandero medicine man (herbalist). We started my six-month apprentice program. For the first month I was permitted only to watch as he worked with his patients. He would almost always give them some peyote tea and herbs of some sort, and then would guide them into an altered state, speaking to them very softly in a deep, hypnotic voice. He would whisper things to them like "this tea will heal you and make you better." (NLP). "I will work with your spirit and mind, the tea and herbs will balance your body and nourish your weak organs."

He was a holistic practitioner in the true sense of the word, which didn't even exist then, or at least I didn't know about it. He would do some very deep massage therapy, sometimes even pop their bones (adjustments). It was sometimes quite brutal, similar to some Rolfing or shiatsu techniques. Other times he would just use imagery to work with their minds. We spent many nights by the fire, listening to him talk about healing and the ways of the spirit-mind, and about how we create illness and how we can die in the digestion and elimination systems. He felt if you can't digest or eliminate properly, you suffer nutritional deficiencies or are flooded with toxins. He was convinced that the mind is responsible for everything. He said if you can think yourself sick, then you can think yourself well. I never understood the power of those statements until many years later.

By 1971 I had been studying healing for six years, and doing massage as well as studying yoga and meditation for about four years. I still knew nothing, yet I thought I knew a lot about healing. Following my return to the States, I continued to study and began to take workshops in Los Angeles. With all the hot, new therapies and nutritional information pouring into the world, I immersed myself in the Holistic Movement. Those were great times. We were fortunate to have spas and clinics like Esalen, the Golden Door, and the Vitoras Institute, which attracted so many great guides for the path to wellness.

I was lucky to have met and studied with some of the greatest healers and teachers of our time. These included the master Buckminster Fuller; Dr. Christopher the herbalist; Bernard Jensen, D.O. iridology and nutrition; Evarts Loomis, M.D.; Dr. John Thie Touch for Health; Dr. Leroy Perry; Ram Dass;, Irving Oyle D.O.; Swami Satchidananda; Elizabeth Kubler Ross; Rolling Thunder; my good friend, Emmett Miller, MD.; Tony Robins and Marshall Thurber, to name a few. Many of you young ones may not have heard of them, but many of my contemporaries haven't either, so don't worry. Educational retreats and workshops on subjects from yoga, nutrition, and spiritual evolution to the "Zen of Tennis" were exploding on the scene. Having read hundreds of books and looking at my work over the previous ten years, I thought that I knew a lot. I still knew nothing; I was still lost in cause and effect.

It wasn't until the mid '70s, when I worked in the clinic and education foundation known as Touch for Health that I felt I started to grow in my profession. At this time I got a lot of experience seeing many patients, and giving lots of lectures and doing workshops. For me, massage was still just a tool to facilitate healing at many levels, and I still had very little control of the results.

Massage: What Does It Really Do?

Let's break it down: It's generally accepted that massage, as we know it, increases the circulation of blood and lymph flow through the body. Massage has a soothing and calming effect on the body and is good for stress reduction. Touch is the most human action: just as a touch on the shoulder is reassuring, just as our mothers' stroking our foreheads and holding us. Touch satisfies the most human need for contact and can be very healing. This kind of contact comes very naturally to some, yet is uncomfortable and awkward for others.

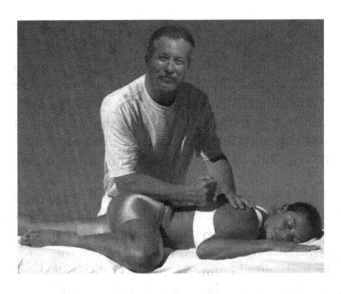

Purpose of Massage

Different types of massage have different purposes. Massage can be used to prevent injuries, or to accelerate healing, as in sports massage, physical therapy, osteopathy, chiropractic, acupuncture, rolfing, etc. What about getting your endorphins going? Massage can sure do that, assisting your brain and glands in secreting chemicals through the body. The effects that these chemicals have on healing are still not fully understood. We are at a crossroads in health and healing. We see that the mind can heal things we thought were out of its jurisdiction or things we considered to be just physical problems. (See Dr. Andrew Weil's *Spontaneous Healing*). The boundaries that we have set up are starting to break down around us.

The AMA has acknowledged and sanctioned acupuncture now because its effectiveness has been supported by science. I find that funny since modern science and modern medicine is only a few hundred years old if we start from the time doctors stopped bleeding people. (Well, before that we accused herbalists, midwives, and other healers of being witches and burned them at the stake. That wasn't too long ago, either.) The use of medicinal herbs goes back 10,000 years, and acupuncture some 5,000 years. I just think that there is something we could learn from these traditional healing systems.

We are all on the same team, and I'm glad to see that natural remedies, nutrition, yoga, and oriental medicine are now part of the mainstream. We all can benefit from the different therapies available to us. Every type of tool or system has a specific healing effect on a specific problem. There is overlap, of course, but basically everything has a purpose and serves an important need. We need communication among all branches of health professions. We need to work together to increase our knowledge and our ability to help our people. We are fortunate to be living in this era of self-awareness, planetary awareness, and body and mind awareness. It can only lead us to greater health, peace and happiness.

OK, so now what do we do? Learn more, right! Like Bucky Fuller said "You can't learn less." Well, now the new saying is "awaken to the greatness that you are!" if we are the center of the universe then we know all there is to know about that center. It's only taking away our own limitations that allow us to be the truth of ourselves.

Helping People

My decades of experience in private practice, in teaching massage therapy, of being a personal trainer and of working in a physical therapy clinic have given me a "training in the trenches" background. Many of my clients were athletes wanting to be better. Some got hurt and later many of my clients had real problems with their bodies, such as ruptured discs, chronic back or neck problems, torn muscles, sprains, cancer, even paraplegia, scoliosis and multiple sclerosis or auto accidents (if there is such a thing as an accident.)

During the late '80s when I was a therapist at Portner's Physical Therapy Clinic, I was frustrated at not being able to get the results I wanted with many chronically injured people. I told myself that I needed to learn more to help these people. At that point, I had been doing massage therapy for close to 20 years. I felt I knew a lot, yet it was not enough. The more I learned about the body-mind connection, the more I felt there was to learn. I taught anatomy, massage, and Kinesiology at the University of Hawaii in Manoa for seven years. I had a massage school and trained more than a thousand students in those 17 years in Honolulu. But I was looking for more--I wanted more out of my therapy. There was something missing. I wanted to learn more, there where a lot of new schools that had home study and I almost did Psychology through Antioch. Dr. Portner told me that I had everything I needed to be a great healer, I didn't have to go back to school and learn more, I knew enough to help the patients I could. I just needed to realize that there where some I could not help and that had to be ok with me.

It was this drive that led me to really look at the body and to ask myself what I was trying to achieve with my work. Let's face it, we cannot diagnose and prescribe with a massage license or even a Ph.D., piled high and deep as they say. Yet we are constantly confronted with the challenge of helping our clients to improve and recover from pain and injury. To really help someone with a muscle problem you need to know anatomy. It is imperative that we understand the mechanics of the body to determine the problem (Kinesiology). Curiously, I have met some therapists who don't want to study anatomy because they prefer to work intuitively. (Can you imagine?).

As I've said before, there are many ways to aid in healing. It's the individual receiving the healing who is ultimately responsible for his or her recovery. We are only facilitators of that restorative energy. The subconscious mind of the receiving person will determine the success of the healing, if there is a subconscious mind. I like to think it's basically our beliefs. In other words, it's our belief structure that we are not victims of the universe that permits the healing whether it's prayer, Indian medicine, acupuncture or just basic mind power. What I realized after all these years and all the techniques is that we should use whatever works. If you don't know how to help someone, pass them on to another practitioner. You both may do the exact same work but get totally different results. Diversity is the beauty of life, so just don't limit yourself with any mind set. Knowledge is worthless if you don't share it, and you can't apply it. You can only live it.

We can assist the healing by working on the body, the mind, nutrition, and the structure, inside out or outside in. I do believe we can heal instantly, but until I have control of that approach or can facilitate that for my clients I have to work with the tools I'm trained to use.

It seems that I have helped many people with pain and problems originating from structural imbalances. It's very gratifying and is the very reason I got into this profession -- to help people. The deepest meaning of any pain or injury goes to the person themselves; they are out-picturing their own struggles.

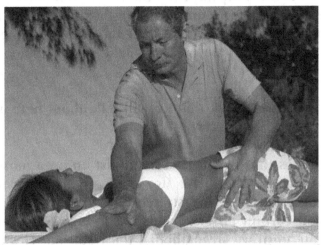

How To Create A New Pattern In The Body

I have put together a system that works to balance the body structurally really, or create another pattern of enhanced wellness. This seems to help people with the basics of dealing with gravity and the imbalances that arise in our bodies due to poor posture, injury, or other factors that cause our bodies to be out of alignment. It's a very gentle, easy stretch. You first go with whatever side is anterior and you follow with the posterior. Now, depending on what side is inferior or superior, you move in the opposite direction with a very gentle stretch of the ligaments. It's not a chiropractic type of adjustment; I don't recommend them unless you are a trained chiropractor.

Keeping it simple is the most difficult part of presenting this work, but I've attempted to succinctly share my discoveries of the last 30 years. I've found that although massage is primarily concerned with the muscles and soft tissue, muscles are not the best avenue by which to achieve balance or to correct structure in the body. We have all heard how the muscles can pull the body out of balance. Yet the more I look at that, having studied Kinesiology, the less I see muscles as the main problem. When working with the theory that the opposing muscle is the problem (George Goodheart or Walter's Kinesiology), we would go around and around the body chasing the problem. In some cases, the more we massaged the muscles, the tenser they became.

When a muscle is out of balance or stressed, the brain shuts it down to prevent further injury. The brain controls all these functions through the propreoceptive nerve reflexes, which make yet another interesting area of study. But are the muscles the cause or the symptom? This question led me to look at the body with different eyes. How can we change the structure to create balance when the hips are rotated or the when one leg is shorter? Or worse, when there is a disc injury or the neck is twisted? How can we permanently correct these problems, create a new pattern for the body, and get the person in touch with what the body is saying?

Massage, chiropractic adjustments, osteopathic consultations, whatever works is how we have approached it. I have seen and worked with some of the best chiropractors in the country and I've witnessed how well it works for some acute conditions, like some locked-facet conditions. But I've come to believe that chiropractic adjustments are not so good for many chronic conditions. If the body has been out of alignment for many years, the quick chiropractic move does not generally produce long-lasting results, nor does it keep the vertebrae or bones in place for long. We can't force the body to change, and if Einstein was right, there is no cause and effect. We can't cause health onto some other body or even our own.

This is just some basic structural work that we will talk about here and just use as a pain relief technique.

Dr. James Cyriax postulates that if you have to adjust an area more than ten times, it's neither the problem nor the solution. I have also seen patients that were over adjusted: they would not stay in, their ligaments were overstretched. Many patients get adjusted and before they're out the door, their chronic physical symptoms return. Sometimes in our P.T. Clinic we would not manipulate until we strengthened the weak muscles and ligaments. These patients did start to get better, but their healings were a much slower process. I found that they stayed properly aligned for a longer time with the slower work.

Deep Muscles of the back

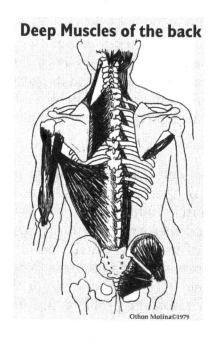

Othon Molina©1979

Bones, Vertebrae & Ligaments

Let's look at the underlying structure of the body: the bones, vertebrae and ligaments. These tissues are not very flexible, and if you've been out of balance for five or ten years, a hard adjustment to these areas may even hurt. But don't get me wrong -- I've seen people improve with regular adjustments, and I've also felt relief after an occasional visit to the chiropractor. Then again, I've also met patients who despite getting adjusted for ten years, they still have back problems.

If you get a quick adjustment, usually the body goes right back to where it was if you even manage to move the bone or vertebra. Ligaments do not respond well to quick movements; they go right back to where they were. When ligaments hold the skeletal structure out of alignment, the body thinks it lives there. If we try to force it to move, it resists. We can try to gently persuade it to move, or loosen it in attempt to align it. If we are out of balance we are constantly having what I call a "muscle tug-of-war." It's a vicious cycle of tension, tight muscles, pain and torque. How do we stop this cycle? One way I know is by balancing the body structurally.

If the deepest level of structure consists of the bones and ligaments, then that's where we can make some long-lasting change. The muscles will follow the bones, as long as the therapist also works on the actual adhesions in the muscle tissues. The way to change the ligaments is through a program of corrective stretches and exercises. We have known in physical therapy that certain corrective exercises can affect postural change in the body, often relieving pain. We also know from sports medicine that in training laying a base is critical. We need to strengthen the muscles, the joints, ligaments, and bones before we put excessive strain on them or we can get injured.

It takes longer to stretch and strengthen ligaments because of their structure, their lack of blood flow, and their rigid cell makeup. Moving ligaments should be a slow and gentle process. Good results require consistency and an accurate knowledge of the structure that you are trying to change. As I have said to many students, the greater your level of knowledge and your diagnostic ability, the more your results will be duplicated. The longer you have treating patients in a clinic day after day, the more you learn about the body and its ability to accept change or resist it. Therapy to me, no matter what type, is still just 60% of the formula for helping people heal their bodies. The other 40% involves a patient's commitment to doing corrective exercises to change the body from within.

During the last ten years I've gotten results in my therapy that I just barely touched on in my first 20 years of work. Many times I heard from patients that I had really helped them, even in the early days. But I couldn't identify what exactly I had done that worked and for years I couldn't always duplicate the results. I always knew that if I worked to balance the body with whatever skills I had, the symptoms or problems would go away or at least improve. It's still a good approach. The key is in our techniques and that determines the level of success. I prefer to work on injury prevention and to help athletes and dancers who want to perform at a higher level. But let's face it: Most patients come to get a massage because they have an existing problem.

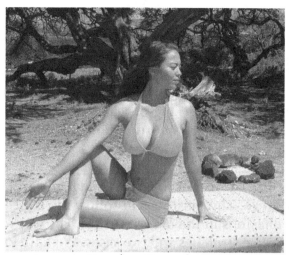

Getting Results

The way I work on the body is with deep massage (for adhesions), DTF (deep transverse friction), and trigger points for the same as well as for increased flexibility, tone, and relief. Then I use positional release techniques holding the area in a stretch, and mobilization techniques using a torque on the whole spine, neck or any joint that I want to work on relaxing. It's a modified version of Orthobionomy that works on the release of the propreoceptive nerve reflexes. This allows the body to release and almost self-align, we persuade it back.

By creating a torque in the spine, for instance, we are persuading the vertebrae and muscles to work as a unit. If we have one that is not cooperating, or is out of alignment, then by applying a fulcrum or a directed force to the area of resistance, we can greatly increase mobility there. I aim the pressure into the direction that the body is being pulled, and then after the body relaxes, I gently coax it back the other way, holding for a few minutes as the patient breathes deeply. This seems to take all the stress off the muscles allowing a deeper relaxation as well as improved alignment.

We use the mechanism of deep respiration, observing the action in the ribs, the undulation of the spine, and movement in the pelvis and the sacrum. These shifts are microscopic, yet they do create movement in the joints. Working with the breath, you can stretch the specific ligament tissue very slowly and gently to achieve restoration and proper alignment in any joints or vertebrae. Notice that we are still working with soft tissue, we are not adjusting bones. It involves very slow and deliberate guidance from your massage therapist.

This system of massage is all within our license. I am not talking about doing any type of chiropractic adjustment nor am I suggesting that we work with the bones. We are addressing soft tissue and using manipulations and stretches with very little force. By prescribing specific stretches to clients that help relieve tension and work toward self-alignment, we encourage the body to change for the better.

The pelvis is the foundation of the body and if it's not balanced, everything has to compensate, usually the muscles of: the legs, the spine, and the neck. If your neck is stressed, rotated or out of alignment, you have constant muscle tension and it can cut your efficiency in energy as well as in movement. People who work at desks or computers all day are prime candidates for neck, low back, and shoulder tension. Sitting and slouching specifically overstretch the posterior ligaments holding the spine together causing weakness, as we don't do enough extension to strengthen them and then they can't support the stress put on them. People sit all day at work then sit in cars driving home for hours, then we sit down to eat dinner, then what do most do is sit and watch TV for hours. This is the dilemma of modern wo/man, and never enough of the right exercises to counter act the sitting and other stresses that gravity imposes.

Most people have rotations in the pelvis and their necks. To ease the pull, I take the neck muscles and massage them first. Then I stretch the neck in the direction it has become accustomed to twist in. So I go with it first to turn off the receptors. Then I bring the neck back and hold it in a stretch to get the tight ligaments and muscles to allow it to go back into place. Using this positional release technique and deep breathing, I have helped people correct their misaligned spines and hips as well as reduce their muscle tension considerably. Then by using my towel techniques I show counteract the pull of gravity with various exercises.

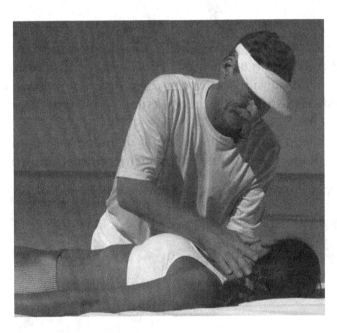

This is my neck alignment technique: I turn the neck following its own torque. Take it further than it is going. Hold for a few deep breaths, then bring to the other direction and hold for a few minutes. This works on the ligaments, and is extremely effective for alignment of the neck.

Since I started really applying these techniques, I have been able to help people that had pain in necks, hips or low back within three or four sessions. Some of these people had been everywhere and had tried lots of therapies including; medication, chiropractic, and had lost hope by the time they came to me. They felt frustrated and were ready for something new. I've seen people change to the point that their hips can stay aligned after four or five sessions, their leg length can stay even, and most importantly, their pain is considerably reduced.

Once patients find something that they can do for themselves, the therapy is part of it. Of course, the ones getting the best results were the ones doing the recommended exercises regularly. Most important for long-lasting results is a commitment to doing the exercises to balance the body.

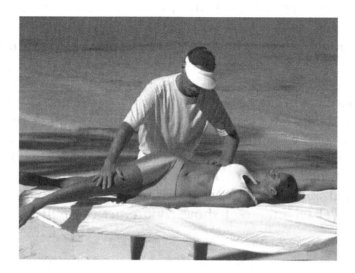

My hip alignment works the same way. Start with the anterior hip, and if superior, take inferior direction and follow with other hip. (Above photo: a superior hip getting stretched inferior.). Never finish with the side that is anterior, or you will leave it more so. The key is to take it where the body is pushing it to, then persuade it back to center.

We can't cause these changes for very long without opening our people to the principle that whatever is going on with their body, it is out-picturing what is going on inside. After all, we are one, are we not?

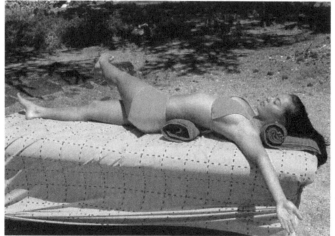

Leilani lengthening the superior hip, and opening the thoracic spine.

This is the self-stretch for the superior hip, it's easy exercises for people to do and they can really help you accelerate their stress reduction via the deeper core alignment. We are working with the ligaments in these very specifically designed exercises. You have to clearly be able to read where they are to design an exercise to get them to improved alignment.

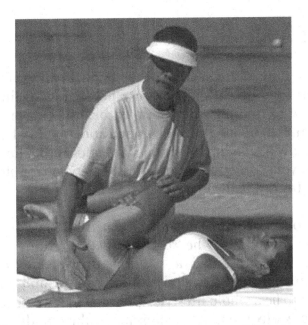

The following is taking the hip that is inferior and stretching it superior, and the gentle approach has always made more sense to me. I am working with very tight structures, the ligaments, which don't really like quick, fast motions. Well, most times they don't. There is a time for hard manipulations or adjustments, just not as often as we have used them, because many chronic conditions do not respond well to them.

Breathing is key in all my work, along with using the imagery and understanding the deeper meaning of what the body is trying to say to you. You get more and more pain sometimes as the body has to speak louder and louder to you. Listen early, and live your life to the fullest and you will not out-picture the struggle that is often masked as pain.

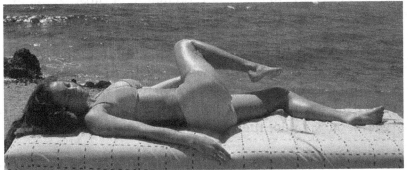

Here Leilani is taking the inferior hip, and stretching superior.

I am teaching these systems in Hawaii and welcome researchers and therapists interested in exploring my work. My other books deal more specifically with full body training and Molina body alignment.

Alignment yoga is the corrective exercise program that I have spent the last ten years refining. It is by no means done; I don't know if I will ever finish all the research into the body. But like everything else in life, it's not the end of the road that's important, but the road itself and living the path daily that gives me the most joy.

Sports Injuries and Micro-Traumas of Athletes

This is more advanced therapy in this section of the book, dealing with most of the common injuries suffered in sports and life. It's about the aches, pains, strains, and sprains that you will encounter from time to time in your therapist or athletic career. Many of these are often minor injuries and heal by themselves without medical help, massage or any treatment. The body is truly a wonderful miracle. Some of these, however, if left untreated can hamper or even end your athletic career, or just give you trouble for years. All this for the love of the sports, or for just being crazy!

Our participation in our own well-being and physical activities is crucial, yet most of us don't have the knowledge of the body to be really effective. Many of the keys to greater knowledge about the body are presented here. I hope to give you the highest level of sports medicine that any therapist, trainer, coach or athlete can use and understand. Because our philosophy is that it's got to be a whole lifestyle approach that we need to use to enhance our lives and well-being. That's why the holistic approach is the one thing pretty much everyone agrees with. So this part of the book is an advanced guide to understanding sports massage, as well as evaluating and treating injuries.

This information is not to take the place of a sports medicine physician. You should always consult with one if you have any doubts. In fact, I find it imperative to have an ongoing relationship with all types of doctors including the orthopedic specialist, osteopathic and physical medicine doctors, an aware chiropractor, naturopath, acupuncturist, and holistic dentist... the works.

We all need to work together. Every discipline serves a purpose and we need all of the different disciplines. They are all vital for our total health because of the different part each plays. Life enhancement is synergistic; working in harmony is the way Nature works best.

This book is intended to give you insight and understanding about several of the most important functions of your body. As well, it will provide an over view of the common and important injuries in athletes or regular clients you may see in a therapeutic clinic, massage practice, or as a trainer or coach. This is equally important for the athlete that wants to be well informed and get the most out of their training program.

Sports massage is primarily concerned with injury prevention. We would rather have our athletes perform better and prevent injuries in the first place. However, as you know elite athletes, as well as most intense people, seem to always push the envelope. With this in mind and after working with executives, athletes and dancers for over thirty years, we need to know effective techniques to assist our patients and ourselves in the healing process.

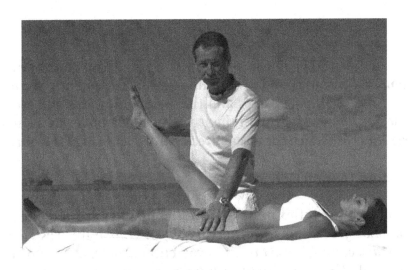

CHAPTER TWELVE
General Testing For Injuries

(See chapters that follow for specific muscle tests.)

Always ask the right questions before doing any testing or evaluations. To test for muscle injury you need to do the following procedure:

1) Hold the joint at mid range and without movement. (A joint held at the extreme end of range could pull the tissues further.) This could hurt, so be careful and always move slowly. If it hurts on a scale of 1-10, 10 being the worst, stop and palpate for the precise injury, and apply appropriate therapy and treatment. If the pain is minimal or not precise enough, continue with next test.

2) Have the athlete contract the muscle being evaluated, starting gradually from a mild contraction to a 75% contraction. If this hurts past a level 6 pain, then palpate for lesion and apply appropriate therapy and treatment.

3) The last resort is to take the muscle through the range of motion very slowly. If the pain is minimal, continue; if it is above 6, stop. Palpate for injury, apply appropriate therapy and treatment. If it hurts in the motion, it could be a ligament.

4) If there is still doubt, do a muscle test or resistance test to the muscle suspected. Pull or push against the action of the muscle. If this causes pain then the muscle being tested has the lesion. Apply appropriate therapy and treatment.

Therapy

Rest, Ice, Compression and Elevation (RICE). For some injuries MICE (movement, ice, compression and elevation) is better. The compression could be compression massage after ice, or if you're trained in wrapping, an ace bandage if it's a serious pulled muscle, which will keep it from swelling further.

Treatment

Deep transverse friction (DTF) is the primary tool used for contractile tissue lesions. (Ligaments and tendons, also respond well to this type of treatment.) We used ice to do the DTF in our clinic. Take small paper cups and fill them with water and freeze. The cup can then be peeled back as you massage with the ice. The paper serves as a slight insulator. We also used large bags of crushed ice for larger areas before applying DTF or compression.

Decreased Circulation: Tension Pain Syndrome

A painful injury can result in reflex muscle contractions and localized muscle guarding. This is common, as the body just wants to protect itself. Of course this restricts movement and local circulation. The swelling is part of the protection as well as part of the problem as it seems to move around. The subsequent ischemia creates more pain. Muscle splinting is intensified and the cycle repeats itself.

This is the vicious cycle that we spoke about earlier. We always found that RICE could break that cycle as well as properly applied massage or trigger point therapy. Trigger point massage with DTF technique is great for releasing the stress or pain within an area.

Pushing or working through the pain results in a more generalized secondary pain area as splinting and the pain cycle begins and moves into other areas. The body can compensate for any trauma. This can then give you other symptoms, which can make it more difficult, so you need to treat the whole person.

Then the secondary more generalized pain area may continue or make the original injury or discomfort worse. Thus it becomes important to treat the original cause as well as the secondary muscle contraction or area of compensation. Massage effectively breaks up these pain cycles by relaxing muscles and increasing the healing process of the body. However, proper massage must be applied for specific injuries, as well as for getting the specific results intended. If you don't know, you won't know what to expect.

Hydrotherapy

This is the use of water in a solid, gas or liquid state to increase circulation and reduce swelling as well as ease muscle tension. These systems have been used for thousands of years. Hippocrates, the father of modern medicine, used water in many ways. And in some very unusual ways, too, like putting water on certain parts of the body for specific maladies. Soaking in mineral baths goes back to the caveman days. We have always used water as a healer and life giver. Just jumping into the ocean has a very healing effect on the body and mind.

Karyokenetic (Ice and Motion: MICE)

In order to reduce the edema as well as regain full functional use of the injured part, ice is used most frequently to anesthetize or numb the injured area, so that some motion is possible (ROM). We would have the patients move the injured area with the ice on them.

Sometimes ankles were put in buckets of ice and then we would have the patient move the foot around. The DTF method for accelerating healing by using the ice cube is of great value at this time as well. Remember, there is a fine line in keeping an injured part of the body immobile, and when you want to keep movement in the area and not have it freeze up on you with improperly formed scar tissue (IFST).

For larger body a part, ice is applied with ice packs, an ice bag, or ice massage (utilizing a large cube of ice and gently rubbing it over the injured area with even, rhythmical strokes). Ice can be applied to smaller parts, such as a foot, ankle, hand or forearm, with an ice bucket or a deep plastic dishpan filled with cold water and crushed or cubed ice.

1. Initially, apply ice for approximately 20 minutes on and 10 minutes off.

2. Passively move the area as long as it remains numb (approx. 3-5 minutes.)

3. Reapply ice until numbness is again reached (approx. 20 minutes.)

4. Repeat movement and Ice for five repetitions, each exercise bout consisting of movement exercises during the numbness (approx. 3-5 minutes). This will reduce the swelling and keep the tissue from forming adhesions.

5. For some injuries in contact sports, we would have the athlete do this all night until they went to bed.

The cold induced numbness is not a total anesthetic, not like an injection of xylocain or lydocain, which some of our doctors used with certain injuries. Ice allows you to have enough sensation, so that if the athlete is over zealous in their exercise, they will feel pain before further injury can occur. All exercise should be performed pain free and should progress as fast as possible from active range of motion (ROM) to weight bearing training and then to full participation in the athlete's sport.

Muscles

Muscles are mostly water and are the motors that move every part of the body. You can't talk, walk, breathe, eat or drink without using your muscles. They all produce movement by the same method, contraction. They pull on their tendons or attachments that in turn move the levers, which are the bones. For example, when the biceps, which is on the front of your upper arm, contracts the forearm, the hand is brought toward your body as in touching your nose. What follows is a description of most of the muscles in the body that we will cover in great detail.

Muscle Soreness

There are all kinds of muscle soreness, which usually sets in eight to twenty-four hours after heavy or unusual exercise. If the pain is very localized, the muscle may be injured to some degree. You may have actually caused some micro-tears in the tissue. However, all muscle soreness is not due to injury alone. If the soreness is diffused, it is probably the result of swelling of the muscle fibers, which are stretched with each muscle contraction. Such soreness is very common, like when you first start weightlifting or working out after a lay off. At those times, I always found some activity or massage on the following day was better than no activity. I would swim and do some stretching or even go on a short bike ride.

Always make sure you are warmed up before stretching. At least break out in a sweat with a slight jog or bike ride first. The only good medical treatment for soreness is a hot tub and some massage. This may help, but depending on the severity it may take some time. Many athletes apply a liniment or take aspirin, but I don't think it does that much. If anything, the aspirin may help.

Even if you are in top physical shape, you can develop soreness in the muscles you don't use often if you are pushing your body. For example, I'm in great shape. I run and I bike. I was skiing cross-country in the winter while living in Oregon for a while. Well, in the winter of 1999 I built some log cabins and did a lot of bending over and lifting logs. Every day I was sore and it took weeks after I finished for the soreness to go away. If you don't use it, you lose it. You can get sore with any new intense activity or in a competition where you push yourself.

Muscle Strain

Muscles when strained can tear and separate. These are called micro-traumas. The problem with these injuries is after they heal they often leave scar tissue, which is not as flexible. So when the athlete goes back to training, it hurts. This is often a time when if the athlete pushes, the area can be re-injured. DTF is especially good during the healing process. It can hurt, so stay within the tolerance level of the athlete. This treatment is especially helpful if the injury is near the origin or insertion of the muscle.

If the injury lies close to the belly of the muscle, the athlete can do some easy movement and non-weight-bearing exercises. Easy biking or swimming in the first few days could be helpful to form a supple scar. If the lesion lies toward the tendon, this approach is less likely to help and DTF must be used. To keep cardio-fitness, I have had runners work their upper body if the injury is in the lower extremities, and the opposite course if needed. Because of the law of reversibility, the first area of training to go is aerobic fitness or conditioning of the lungs and heart.

Muscle Pull

A pulled muscle is an acute tear of muscle fibers and is characterized by sudden, localized, and persistent sharp pain in a muscle that is being stressed. The sprinter gets it in the hamstring, the swimmer and baseball player in the shoulder, and the football player just about anywhere. Even though there are more than four hundred major muscles, very few of them are actually ever injured. It's just a small handful that is normally hurt.

When a muscle starts to tear, it will really hurt. When you develop a sudden, sharp pain in a muscle, stop exercising immediately. If you attempt to continue exercising, you will cause further damage to the muscle fibers and prolong the healing time. I have heard hamstrings actually pop quite loudly.

A muscle pull is not much different than a strain; it's just more serious and intense. The muscle and or tendon may have torn, and that creates a similar situation only with more swelling and tissue death. The treatment is much the same: RICE, DTF and rest are critical. Never stretch the pulled muscle or use longitudinal massage strokes directly on it. Also, stay away from resistance exercises; both of these are contra indicated during this period. Those muscles which are most likely to benefit from therapeutic movement during the first few days are the quadriceps, hamstrings, gastrocnemius, gluteus, biceps, pectoralis major, latissimus dorsi, and trapezius.

Any other muscle pull can become potentially more injured with movement including the groin, abdominal, and neck muscles as well as some of the major tendons in the arms and legs. (See specific testing of injured areas later in the book)

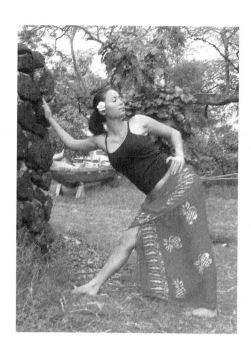

CHAPTER THIRTEEN
General Causes for Muscle Pulls

Muscle pulls result when more tension or stress is applied to a muscle than it can handle. As a general rule, the more intense and sharp the pain, the more extensive the injury. Muscles that have not been warmed-up are most often the ones pulled. Cold muscles are stiff and tight and susceptible to injury. In the old days, football players hardly stretched; now it's one of the largest parts of their conditioning. Stretching prevents many of the injuries to muscles. Not warming up right is a problem only outside of the professional teams and competition. Well, maybe it includes the Olympic level athlete as well. For many runners, their idea of stretching is leaning on the lamppost for a few minutes and then taking off running. Well, maybe not as true nowadays. We have been in the jogging revolution for over twenty years, and there is enough information out there for the weekend warrior. But do you follow it? That's what's important; you have to do what works best.

Any intense athletic activity at most levels without warm up causes all kinds of muscle pulls as well as more acute musculo-skeletal problems. Even something as simple as stretching has become a whole science now.

What-to-do information is flooding us, but very little information about what not to do is available. The key is proper stretching, and it's vital for everybody. Before playing a sport or running, you should warm up for at least ten or fifteen minutes by performing easy running or biking with slow, easy movements. Then stretch and gradually increase the pace in training.

Poor flexibility, not enough stretching in your program or not building the proper base in your training program will cause muscle pulls. Think of this: Every time you exercise hard, your muscles are slightly damaged (micro-trauma). With healing they shorten, and like a tight string they are more susceptible to tearing, unless you have restored flexibility by stretching and lengthening the body. Flexibility is one of the most important components in injury prevention. This is achieved through stretching and massage. There is no other way. Swimming might create some flexibility, but most muscle activity is through contraction.

Poor flexibility can cause an imbalance between the sides of the body, the muscles or a joint. This could inhibit full range of motion (ROM) during the heat of competition. We push the body beyond its capacity with a certain activity or specific action. During the competition, athletes attempt to run their fastest, jump higher, lift the most, throw harder, and so on. Many will hurt themselves because they are on endorphins (the body's morphine) that produce that "natural high," as well as many histamines and natural hormones. Flexibility and stretching pays off. If supple enough, there is no muscle tug-of-war and there will be less chance of injury. That's if you don't fall, crash, slip, drop the weights, etc.

Flexibility is very specific to each person and their body type as well at to each specific body part that we are dealing with. Ligament stability is within the joint and these are not very flexible (see ligaments section). If they are torn, there is a great risk of injury and even surgery could be needed.

Flexibility is important for maintaining joint stability and preventing aging and injury, as well as for increased athletic performance.

Strength plus flexibility equals speed. This is a formula I have used for years to explain the importance of stretching and massage for athletes. Stretching programs should be started gently and slowly, never going into pain, as overstretching can lead to injury.

Over training also causes muscles pulls. Every time you exercise intensely, your muscles suffer slight damage (micro-trauma). If you exercise intensely again before your muscles have had time to heal, you are much more likely to injure them further. Most injuries are caused by over training, insufficient or no real warm up, and not stretching well. This adds to poor flexibility, muscle imbalances, mineral deficiency, out of alignment structure, improper base-building or inadequate endurance. Many runners used to just run many miles a week. I knew many doing upwards of ninety miles. That's just too much on any body. Now they know more about interval training, cross training, and getting massage. The specificity law in training always applies (see Natural Laws of Training).

Some of the damage is usually from hemorrhaging in the tissue. It's just like pounding your leg with a two-by-four! That's what I used to tell those runners back in the '70s. Now we know that there is also enzymatic and metabolic as well as leukocyte buildup in the tissues. Basically, what happens is that you bleed a little internally from micro-trauma, tears to the muscle fibers. You release more toxins as you exercise and burn more calories, and you increase the heat in the whole body. This takes you into high overload. Properly monitored, this is how you must train. But without the proper knowledge, you can also tear down the body. With awareness you can help the body heal itself faster. When we increase the demands on the body, this causes stress and stretch. This is what is experienced by the muscles, ligaments, and other systems all of which compounds the problem.

Over training is very often found in long to middle distance runners, weightlifters, and professional triathletes. The elite athlete competing just statewide these days is in a very demanding position. Many weightlifters get injuries as well, because to be competitive in that arena you have to push. Even just weightlifting for your sport, football, basketball, baseball, track, triathlons... heck, almost every sport but chess needs weight training. My feeling is almost everybody needs to weight lift, or have a very sophisticated strength-training program.

So to be highly successful again, you have to be exercising two times a day, six days a week. Some even do it seven days a week (which I don't recommend). In strength training, there is an alternate, intermittent stress placed on a tendon and muscles. This makes the size of the muscle and tendon to grow, helping to build the strength and integrity of the attachment. Since the origin is an attachment is immovable, proximal on the trunk, or nearest the trunk. The insertion is usual the furthest away, or distal. The origin and insertion are rarely on the same bone. In weightlifters, the tendon may become so enlarged that it will not stay in its proper groove or place, e.g., the biceps tendon will fall out of the bicepetal groove sometimes. Shoulder problems are very common, and therapy does not help very much. Exercise is far more important for the shoulder than anywhere else.

The over training syndrome begins with feeling flat emotionally, kind of not caring much about anything except for training, because of the intense addiction that happens with a compulsive, highly competitive athlete. Many corporate executives are just as intense, and if they happen to be high corporate elite athlete, hold on to your jock strap! You have a lot to handle. That's part of the mental aspect that we cannot overlook. This tends to create a metabolic build up in the muscles with no recovery time as well. Muscles can't stand this type of trauma with so much frequency and not enough rest.

Be careful, however, in explaining all this to the athlete. They mostly want to know "how bad am I hurt, how long rehab will take, and when can I start training again" The worst thing that can happen is getting re-injured by starting to train too soon or intensely. Sometimes talking about yoga or stretching programs even meet with some resistance, because of the time crunch. Like an athlete saying "what? Stretch before and after a run, for at least an hour a day?" The comeback: "Jesus, I don't have time to stretch, I can't possibly fit it into my day." Or in telling them to train less, just once a week to take a day of rest. I would then say, "Now, since you really don't need to train so much you can stretch in its place." Thus the law of hard and easy days came to be. (See laws of training.)

5. Muscle imbalance is another source of pulled muscles. Every muscle that moves a joint in one direction has an opposing muscle that moves it in the opposite direction (the antagonist). One muscle acts as an antagonist to the other and will often be stronger, placing the balance of stress on the joint capsule. We are just like lever and pulley machines. We are a walking moving structure and these physical principles have nothing to do with belief or philosophy, this is science.

It's a common problem with the quads and the hamstring group. The quadriceps group is twice as strong as the hamstring group, so consequently the majority of injuries happen to the hamstrings in running sports (See other sports injuries). A basic muscle imbalance between the quadriceps and hamstrings can also be a cause of cramps and muscle spasms, causing problems with running. If you have a client with a powerful quadriceps, I would suggest having them put twice the effort in training the hamstrings to help balance it. Correction can only happen by strength training the hamstring; it's the only way. There will always be an imbalance anyway, as the quadriceps is usually much stronger. You can bring this down to 1 1/4 times as strong by strengthening.

This has to be done with all of the major muscle groups. Not only is this critical to athletes, it's just as important for sedentary people. Gravity is our worst enemy and it's the cause of most of our physical stress. This is a key aspect of using applied Kinesiology for balancing the body to assist in improved performance and reduced aches and pains.

Water or mineral deficiency cause pulled muscles. Again, because of the demand on the body, the heat from muscle action, the increase in toxin and free radicals, and all the stuff that happens when you turn up the volume. The body uses up more nutrients as well. Vitamin C, magnesium, phosphorus and calcium are the important components of muscle contraction. Twitching, spasms, and some pain all come from lack of these minerals. A charley horse is a blow to the thigh or quadriceps, characterized by intra-muscular bleeding. A charley horse is not a cramp or a spasm (see stitch.)

If the problem is a mineral imbalance, fluid intake is critical especially in the warmer climates. NOT orange juice, it's too sweet, but most citrus juices are great if you water them down. Sometimes electrolyte drinks can greatly help this condition, so try other fruit juices or a sport drinks. The key is that they have less than 5 to 10% sugar. Lack of water, again, is the usual cause for cramps, but it's good to add the mineral replacement for the long run. There are really good electrolyte drinks at the health food stores.

Structural abnormality is also a source of muscle pulls. Although this is not too often a reason, certain structural abnormalities, such as flat feet, unequal leg length, or a deep curve in the back (lordosis) have the effect of putting excess stress on a particular muscle and make that muscle more likely to be injured. Lordosis can cause undue stress on the hamstrings, or abdominals, and low back pain is a common injury to most people, not just athletes.

Structural balance is an important emphasis for athletes. I'm talking about more subtle discrepancies than bone length, leg length. Most humans have a rotated hip, some sacral or lumbar rotation, and many upper thoracic or neck misalignments. This is not theory. I have seen thousands of bodies, and even some Olympic athletes have imbalances. Just think what the muscles have to do, over the years either through functional habits, injuries, or from what just plain life has laid on us. We have the muscles playing tug-of-war. Most of us have this as well, a discrepancy that may look structural. However, if the bones are found to be the same length, then it's a soft tissue (muscle, tendon or fascia) problem. Structural massage and a holistic exercise program are needed to correct this. Not only can the misalignment cause injury, but the body is also functioning at a very inefficient level. It sometimes takes the involvement of many more muscles than are needed to perform an action. This wastes energy as well, not to mention what it does to the whole nervous and propreoceptive system.

All training programs should include gradual increases in workload, speed, and resistance. It's important to build a solid foundation, for any athletic endeavor. You have to know what you are doing or get good expert advice on a training program. I ran personal and corporate training programs for many years. I also worked with a number of elite, teams, dancers, and athletes. Rapid increases in these structural factors often lead to more stress than a muscle can handle and results in an injury. It's best to get a full orthopedic and muscle evaluation and have a building program tailored for your specific body needs and goals in sports before competing or heavy training.

Trauma or injury by blow is another source of injury to muscles. Stepping into a hole, twisting your ankle or being hit by someone can cause muscle damage and consequent injury to the tissue. Being hit, thrown, jumped on or having direct intense pressure to a particular body part, twisting a leg, a knee, or throwing 90 miles-an-hour for a baseball game can all hurt your body in different ways. We also have car accidents in this category of contact sports injuries. RICE immediately to all injuries and sports massage for rehabilitation are the best techniques to aid in the healing. Stress fractures are usually caused by impact over a long period of time, as well as weak muscles not capable of handling the shock absorption quality of the muscle action. These can be treated with the same program but the most important part in stress fractures is structural.

The lack of an adequate foundation can cause pulled muscles. The proper endurance-building program is very important. Sustained, rhythmic endurance exercises thicken the muscles, tendons, and ligaments and make them more resistant to injury. In the old days, it was called LSD for long, slow distance to build up the tissues. Most competitive athletes train all year now; they just time their peak for their completion events.

The athlete's musculature problems, as we said earlier, are mostly the micro-traumas that occur because they have not built a good running base for the miles they are attempting to compete in. Many times athletes need some good advice as well as massage and soft tissue manipulation. Always stay within your realm of knowledge and license. If you can't help them, refer them to someone else. We can do so much within our massage license; so don't be stepping on others' toes. Let's create a network of professionals. We have enough injured people to go around. Know who to recommend and when to recommend your client to another therapist.

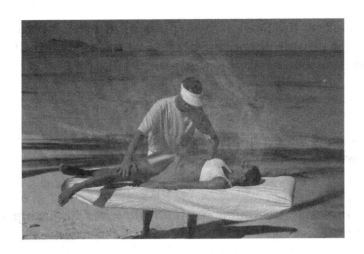

CHAPTER FOURTEEN
Assessment and Treatment of Sports Injuries

The greatest contribution massage therapists can make to athletes is in rehabilitation and the prevention of soft tissue injuries. It is critical to teach the athlete about stretching, cross training, and proper body mechanics. It also helps the athlete to get regular treatments and stay limber, balanced, and in tune. Constant stretching, proper nutrition, and proper corrective body alignment exercises besides proper training are critical to staying competitive. Once the athlete is injured, then the proper evaluation and treatment plan is necessary. It doesn't matter whether it's a micro-trauma from over use or larger lesions from more traumatic injuries. It's critical to know what to do, and most importantly, what not to do.

Massage is a valuable tool as an adjunctive treatment for both chronic and acute injuries. The clinical use of massage has increased a lot since I first got into it. There are many medical clinics that have a massage therapist on staff now.

Training is most important because we have to be aware that massage improperly administered or the use of the wrong type of technique can worsen acute injuries. If in doubt, refer to a qualified sports medicine doctor or sports massage specialist.

Always refer a serious injury to a doctor, and if you have the qualifications and a relationship with the doctor there is no reason why he will not refer the athlete back for massage. I always felt that if it's your client, even referring them to another more qualified massage therapist that you know and respect is ultimately helping the client most. That massage therapist would honor your relationship, and the client would honor and respect you. There is no ethics in taking clients from anyone; there are plenty of people to go around.

Most physicians and trainers recommend the use of heat for forty-eight hours after the pull has occurred. We continue with ice as long as there is pain. Heat dilates the blood vessels and increases the blood supply, which brings increased amounts of nutrients to the injured area. We sometimes used ice and heat after forty-eight hours or longer, depending on the injury and the results from the prior treatment administered. Nutrients are the muscle's building blocks and also provide energy for healing. Massage is one of the best therapies for long term healing and nutrient increase in the tissue.

General Assessments

We will look closer at each muscle in following chapters. Pain is usually the main key to any assessment at the gross level.

Pain

Massage may be an effective treatment for pain, however done improperly can tend to create more pain regardless of its cause.

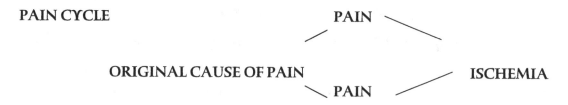

PAIN CYCLE

PAIN

ORIGINAL CAUSE OF PAIN   ISCHEMIA

PAIN

Cryostretch

During cryostretch, both ice and stretching are utilized to decrease muscle spasms. Exercises consist of a combination of static stretching (passive) and the contract-relax technique of propreoceptive neuromuscular facilitation (active PNF).

A. Initial ice application for approximately 10-15 minutes

B. Cryostretch exercise:

1. Therapist passively stretches the muscle by moving the affected limb until the athlete begins to feel tightness and/or pain. Movement with the ice for most injuries is very important.

2. Therapist holds the limb in that position for 8 to 15 seconds.

3. Athlete actively contracts the affected muscle for 5 seconds. Begin slowly and builds up to an 85% contraction. Therapist provides resistance so that the limb does not move.

4. Athlete relaxes the contraction. Therapist moves the limb until the athlete feels tightness and/or pain (ROM will be greater here than it was in step 1). Hold for 10 seconds.

5. Repeat steps 2, 3, and 4 twice more. (i.e., contract-relax-move limb and hold - Contract-relax-move limb and hold.)

6. Complete three bouts of exercise with applied numbness in between each bout (reapplying ice for approximately 3-5 minutes). Each exercise bout consists of two 60-second repetitions of static stretch - static contraction; with a 20 second rest in between.

Secondary Muscle Spasm

A healthy muscle will function without pain or weakness. The pain needs to be measured during inactivity, movement, walking or the motion that hurts the most, and last of all, in resistance. Manually applied tension to an injured muscle will result in increased pain. This should be done last and very carefully. I've always found palpation and asking the athlete questions is very effective in assessing an injured muscle. This is the reason why Kinesiology is so critical in a massage therapy or an orthopedic evaluation. If you know the muscle and you know the movement, you can often determine the injured muscle by the action that causes pain.

The tissues that massage is concerned with are contractile or inert. Contractile tissues are muscles, tendons, and their attachments to the bone, whereas inert tissues are ligaments, joint capsules, bursa, and fascia. These inert tissues move with the joints, and because they lack blood and have dense cell structure, they are slower to heal. The way to test for injury in these tissues is by an orthopedic examination, checking the range of motion (ROM), or putting a stretch on the ligament by pulling on the joint at the affected site. A word of caution here: Be very careful with serious injuries, and if you are not qualified to evaluate, refer the patient to a competent doctor. Passive joint movements are the safest way to assess these inert tissues first. (Remember, we don't diagnose or prescribe, but we must determine the area we are to work on).

Whereas resisted movements are used to assess contractile muscle and tendon tissues, as massage therapists our concern will be primarily with resisted movements. This is why I always stress Kinesiology for massage therapists. If you can't determine what muscle is injured, you can't help as effectively.

Just as important, if you don't know the right type of massage for the particular injury, you not only won't help much, you can make it worse.

This goes for healthy athletes: I have seen massage therapists give too deep and too intense a massage to a new patient before a race, and the athlete can't perform as well. If they are not used to deep massage, that is certainly not the type of treatment to be given before a competitive event.

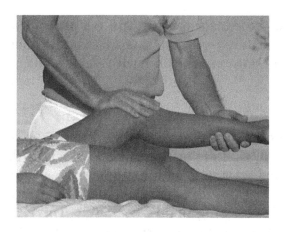

CHAPTER FIFTEEN
Resistance Testing Muscles

A hamstring pull is treated in the same manner whether it occurs in a football player, a dancer or a runner. For each of the six internal tissue structures of the body (muscles) most frequently involved in sports injuries, the same principles apply.

To accurately assess muscle, tendons, and ligaments attachments to bone, the therapist will examine for pain and/or weakness. Weakness here can be relative. If you have worked with the patient before or they are very in tune with their body, they will say "I feel weak when you do that." If the tissue is strong and painless, there is no problem. If the tissue is weak and painless then there are possible nerve conduction problems or propreoceptive nerve imbalances. Refer this to a doctor if you suspect serious injury. If the tissue is more painful while being stressed with a resisted movement, a lesion probably exists.

It's important to apply the resistance in the exact opposition to the muscle being evaluated for accuracy. After that, palpation for accurate location of the lesion is critical. Apply appropriate therapy and treatment plan.

Tendons

Tendons are strong fibrous bands that attach muscles to bone; they are not flexible like muscle. To understand better what a tendon is, find the wide part of your calf muscle in the middle part of the back of your lower leg. The tendon starts where the wide calf muscle suddenly becomes a narrow band above your heel. This is your Achilles tendon. With your hand, follow the band down to where it attaches to the back of your heel bone. This will give you an idea of how hard tendons are.

Muscles and tendons are very similar, they only differ a bit in their cellular composition. Tendons, which are rope-like extensions of the muscles, do not contract; only muscles cells do. For example, when the calf muscle contracts, it pulls the Achilles tendon up which in turn pulls the foot down (plantar flexion). When muscles are shortened by hard exercise, the tension of the muscle -tendon complex is increased. Thus, there is the need for stretching before and after exercise.

Tendons are more susceptible to injury than muscles for two reasons. Tendons have a smaller cross section than muscles do. That means they don't have as large or as wide an area over which force can be distributed. As a result, there is more strain on most tendons than on muscles during exercise. Also, tendons are located in areas where they can be injured easily, usually at the origin or insertion of the muscles. They are located at the attachment points and some have no sheath or protection. On the other hand, muscles are located in protected areas. They rarely rub against other rough tissue and have more padding (fat and fascia).

Tendon Rupture

A tendon rupture is a separation of a tendon from a bone or muscle, or a complete tear in the tendon itself. THIS IS UGLY! and causes very serious, major PAIN. Muscle separations are the most common tendon ruptures, but it does happen at the bone, too. Send to a doctor immediately.

Common Causes for Tendon Rupture

Tendon ruptures are usually the result of sudden, violent contractions. They occur most often in sprinters, football players, weightlifters, and athletes in other sports where sudden bursts of speed are required. Athletes who are tight, inflexible, and are not properly conditioned, or have not warmed up their muscles are obviously most susceptible to tendon ruptures.

When an athlete ruptures his tendon, you generally can hear a loud pop. The pain is so severe that the athlete usually screams in pain and holds the affected muscle in a contracted position. I once saw an athlete tear his rectus femoris at the origin. It created a huge ball of muscle on his thigh. This is a very severe injury. He would not let anyone touch it or be moved. Usually they won't even let it be examined unless they first receive pain medicine. The athlete was carried off on a stretcher to a doctor. If a tendon rupture is suspected, consult a physician immediately. In the meantime, apply RICE.

The area over the tendon becomes swollen and usually hurts for days. After a day or two, a huge black and blue mark from the internal bleeding appears on the skin overlying the rupture. By sending out fibrous filaments into the surrounding tissue, tendons sometimes can reattach themselves within a couple of weeks. The best way to prevent recurrences after it has healed is to stretch the tendon daily and get treatments of DTF. After it has healed, a good stretching and balancing program needs to be implemented.

Ruptured Achilles tendon

In sports that require running, the Achilles tendon is ruptured far more commonly than most any other tendon in the body. Ruptures of other tendons are rare and are usually the result of an unnatural force or extreme force. However in power lifting there seem to be more tendon injuries because of the extreme weights being used. For example, when a weightlifter slips in an action, he can tear a tendon in a leg, an arm or a wrist.

A tendon rupture is very serious, and there are times it becomes a medical emergency, as when the tendon tears too far away from its attachment site so that it can't reattach itself on its own. There are also times when a piece of the bone is torn off with the tendon. In both of these conditions, it may be necessary to sew or staple the tendon back with surgery.

A strain to a tendon also results in a tearing of fibers. Each time the muscle connected to the tendon contracts, there is further tearing. This results in an inflamed hematoma and swelling. It will then form scar tissue and it will get worse if not treated. The scar tissue can be eliminated with DTF, and you can use the ice cube in the acute stages. I found that DTF does not feel that great, even when there is no injury, so go easy. Read the works of Dr. James Cyriax. I was fortunate to train and study with a doctor that used these methods of DTF and believed in Dr. Cyriax's work, Dr. Bernard Portner in Honolulu, Hawaii.

Ligaments

Ligaments are tough fibrous bands that attach to the ends of the bones as they meet to form the joint. Their main function is to hold the bones together when the joint moves. They are not at all flexible and have very little blood supply, so they heal very slowly.

Ligaments can hold the bones together so tightly that there is very little movement of the joint. Like the vertebrae in your spine, they can move only slightly. Ligaments can also be flexible enough to allow a wide range of motion. Good examples of mobile joints are those of the extremities - the shoulders, the most mobile joint, hips, knees, ankles, toes, wrists, fingers and the elbows.

If some of the fibers of the ligament are torn, it is called a sprain. To avoid further tearing of these fibers, the joint should be immobilized immediately. Of course, RICE will help. If all of the fibers are torn, the injury is called a complete ligamentous rupture. In most cases, the ligament reattaches itself by laying down new cells, but sometimes surgery will be needed if the tear is severe.

All joint injuries, whether they involve bones, cartilage, ligaments, or the muscles and tendons that attach near the joint, have the potential to end an athletic career.

If you incur an injury to a joint whether it is your shoulder, elbow, wrist, finger, toe, ankle, knee, or hip, treat it immediately with RICE. Never exercise or stretch a joint that has just been injured. If the pain or swelling is severe or lasts beyond forty-eight hours, seek help from a sports medicine doctor.

I realize that in most cases the pain will not be gone in forty-eight hours, and as a result many people will be seeing their doctors unnecessarily.

However, the diagnosis and management of joint injuries requires special training that cannot be taught in a book. So, I would rather send you to a doctor needlessly rather than taking a chance that you will not receive the proper diagnosis and treatment for a potentially serious problem.

A ligament that is overstretched (sprain) results in pain, just as with the other tissues. Ligaments will hurt more with passive movement and ROM of the injured area. Also, most of the time ligaments will hurt under weight bearing or walking. They feel hot, cold or sharp pain and it seems to be more localized than muscle injuries. While healing, the ligament can become attached to adjacent muscle or bone, creating less mobility and adhesions. DTF moves the ligament in imitation of its natural movement and stops it from adhering to adjacent muscle and bone.

In fact, DTF aids all adhesions whether they are new or old. Old injuries just take longer. Acute injuries heal much faster with DTF and ice, and that can be used effectively for the first week to ten days. NO HEAT EVER ON INJURIES (even after forty-eight hours, especially if there is still pain, we don't recommend heat at all even though most others say use heat after forty-eight hours).

Joints and Cartilage

A joint is the place between two bones that functions like a hinge so that the bones can move in relation to each other. Some don't have much movement. The ribs, skull bones, and the spine all have minimal movement compared to the other joints.

Cartilage, a tough, white gristle that contains hardly any blood vessels or nerves, lines the ends of the bones of a joint and protects the bones from rubbing against each other. If a cartilage is broken or chipped, the end of the bone is unprotected, and the bone can gradually wear down from friction against the cartilage of the opposing bone. Each movement will be painful because the end of the unprotected bone contains a rich supply of nerves.

A common injury is cartilage damage to the knees, often called torn cartilage that can come from hits as in football or other sports, or twists to the knees that occur in falls, skiing, etc.

Fasciae

Fasciae are the strong, thick white fibrous sheets that surround, protect, and support almost all the tissue in the body: muscles, tendons, joints, nerves, blood vessels, and organs. Fascia looks and feels to some degree like ligaments and tendons and contains the same four components: two types of fibers, fluid, and connective tissue cells.

In athletes, fasciae absorb some of the pressure on tendons, muscles, and joints, and help protect them from injury.

The Skin

The skin is the largest organ in the body. It is our outermost covering and consequently is at high risk of being damaged, injured, and infected. It keeps us together, literally holding all the muscles and organs inside. It also helps to keep us warm and cool. It is amazing how well the skin stands up to a constant attack of germs, dirt, pollution, scrapes, bangs, friction, sun, wind, heat, and cold. There are reasons your skin lasts so long and stays in fairly good shape:

133

It's constantly replacing itself with new cells; the old ones fall off as new ones are produced. You grow a new surface layer of skin every twenty-eight days or so. If you cut yourself, the skin will grow up to seven times faster to repair itself.

It is specially adapted in many ways to resist infections. It maintains a dry outer surface, which prevents germs and bacteria from forming. Wetness provides an environment that frequently leads to germ or bacterial growth. Many problems with skin or bacterial infection can be helped just with sun and saltwater, or by jumping in the ocean. It also can protect itself from intense use: If skin is frequently and vigorously rubbed, as occurs in manual labor or many sports, it will protect itself by forming a thick covering called a callus. The skin can adapt to many environments.

This is the major organ we deal with in massage, as well as what's under it. All the soft tissue is our domain. Learn it well. Following are most of the muscle groups that we work with in massage therapy.

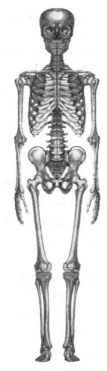

CHAPTER SIXTEEN
The Spine & Neck

The spine is very strong, and since it has taken thousands of years of evolution for the body to develop to where we are, it's amazing that it can still be a source of trouble. I think most of us have had some kind of back or neck problem during our life. If you haven't, you're lucky; it can be a real pain. Most of us know someone who has suffered back problems of one kind or another. We hear of sciatica (pain shooting down the leg or in the buttocks) being mentioned often, or a slipped disc, and then again we hear "I threw my back out." All three of these expressions are rather medically incorrect and misleading terms. We'll go into detail about what this all means.

The bones of your spine are called vertebrae. They are stacked one on top of the other. The spine changes shape, tapering down and out from top to the bottom. It's our support column and without it we would have no structure. It along with the cranium holds the nervous system, the spinal cord, and nerves. The spine is actually composed of some 26 irregular bones that create a strong grid with some flexibility to allow movement.

The spine supports the whole body and can take tremendous stress. Up to 1,200 pounds or more of pressure can be absorbed by just the discs. Discs are the shock absorbers between the vertebrae. The disc is made up of two kinds of cartilage, a hard outer layer and a soft, spongy, jelly type center. These discs give your back the shock absorbent qualities and the resilience to shock and stress that can be put on the spine.

Treating disc injuries varies greatly. Depending on how they came on will determine the treatment. There just doesn't seem to be any definitive way to treat some of them at times since they can be as different as people are. Massage or manipulation seems to bring relief.

In some cases proliferant injections to strengthen the ligaments surrounding the disc are helpful if they are weak or hyper mobile. Traction can either bring relief or make you worse, usually in acute stages. When pain is severe, an injection can be given into the nerve, which completely deadens the nerve being pinched by the disc. This is called a nerve block, or an epidural. In some cases, surgery to remove the disc is recommended. These last two treatments are the extreme cases included just to give you the range of treatments that are available.

Sometimes just good old "doctor time" and this amazing body takes care of itself. Often the protruding portion of the disc is said to dry up and is reabsorbed by the body, thus releasing the pressure on the nerve. However, this can take as much as nine months to a year, and depending on how you go at life, you could have it again soon if you don't address the core issue.

That means if you have gotten it from over use syndrome which means that your bad posture got you there, then if you continue with the bad posture you will stress the area again. Contrary to some beliefs, discs can get weaker after several injuries, not stronger as bones do. If the problem is the ligaments are too stretched, then sometimes sclorosing can help if they are brittle from injuries, or if you have been in a severe accident. Either way, depending on the injury, the primary cause of the injury, along with the inherent weaknesses of the structure of this particular individual will determine the best short term as well as the long term treatment and educational program to follow. Some exercises are great but not to be done during the acute phase. Others will help greatly when done early, and then later for strengthening and prevention of injuries. These many disciplines need to work synergistically, and when you have several components missing, well, you miss the mark. Nonetheless, you will help the body more by using the appropriate tools and timing.

There are many disciplines that are important constituents of the process. For example, any stress on the body, physically as well as mentally, creates a certain physiology in the body. These many conditions were brought out by Dr. Hans Selye, the man who coined the word "STRESS," when he said that stress caused about 65-75% of illnesses. Mind-induced muscle tension is almost like having a pulled muscle that happens over a long period of time. This is the over use syndrome that I refer to. As you stress that muscle, it has to use histamines as a way of reaching homeostasis. Blood flow could be restricted, and toxins then build up when the body over uses its natural resources or chemicals, including, cortisone, anti-inflammatory histamines, and endorphins (the body's own pain medication).
The irritation from this overworked muscle swells, creating a weaker muscle condition chemically and mechanically. Now it's structural as well.

We don't know what comes first: mental, physical, or structural. The funny thing is, I think it can come from any direction. "Why" doesn't' matter only as much as to know what to do, when to make it all better faster, and more effective. We need to assist the body, not take over the direction we think it should go.

So all of this leads you to a necessary understanding of the conditions and the systems and best tools applied at the appropriate time. RICE, of course, is always the best medicine. There comes a time when the body may need a natural anti-inflammatory tool (Wobenzime

N is great) when its own are taxed, and these are available from massage, acupuncture, or any therapy, all the way up to medicines and injections.

What's important to understand is that even with these treatments, there is a time when they work well, and a time when they are no longer effective. All conditions being the same, we could have some rules and laws about healing, and often you hear even medicine is not an exact science. There is a factor we call art, but you could also call it common sense. The thing is, for every law and rule I have always found one or more exceptions. So if there is an exception, it cannot be a law or truth. We have to treat and work with each individual, each circumstance, and the specific set of events to be more effective.

Ultimately, it's all dependent on the individuals to heal themselves as it always points to lifestyle and how you live your life. So that leads me to approach all of it looking at the whole, not the parts, as well as using all the tools available to us.

Each vertebra is held in place by hundreds of ligaments that criss-cross from vertebra to vertebra in a very complex structure. Each vertebra has two bony transverse protrusions like wings, and a third one called the spinous process that is in the posterior part of the vertebra. This part of the vertebra at the rear protects the spinal cord. There are holes in the middle of the vertebrae and these holes line up together and form a long tunnel. This is where the spinal cord and its nerves are located. The nerves exit out from the spinal cord through an opening on each lateral side of the vertebra. It's at this exit that we have the basic problem with discs pressing on the nerve. It's usually discs pressing on nerves that cause the condition we call back pain, or sciatica. Sometimes due to a strain, injury, lifting something too heavy or a car accident, you may also injure the ligaments. These ligaments can also be torn with over use of the back or long time stress.

I can't tell you how many times I've heard a patient say, "I just bent down to pick up a newspaper and, wham, I threw my back out." I could buy a new house if I had a buck for all the times I heard this, or "I was brushing my teeth, I coughed, and my back went out." I think about 80 to 90 %t of people in the world have back or neck problems, or maybe confined more to the United States and other modern countries. (I think there are fewer back problems in the third world countries.) The statistics say fewer, one out of three, but I'm not sure that's right. Anyway, most back and neck problems relate to injuries to some part of the spine complex, either the soft tissue (muscles or ligaments) or the discs themselves.

There are over 48 major nerves that come out of the spine. The nerves are the network for the communication between the brain, the nervous system, organs and the rest of the body. There is a lot of controversy about the spine and back problems. It's a very mysterious part of the body because it is so complex.

There are many misconceptions about the back, its pain and its treatment. Because it really takes a doctor or therapist who has experience with the back to understand the problem, many general practitioners may not always agree or have a clear diagnosis as to what is going on. First, there are many similar symptoms that can come from different problems, as well as many types of treatments for the many injuries. Knowing which treatment and when to use it is the key to improving the patient's condition. This is where the experience of seeing hundreds of back pain patients comes in.

The Spine and Its Structure

In my opinion, the spine is one of the most fascinating parts of the body. If you look at the spine you find that the bones are very odd shapes. They're smaller at the top and get larger towards the bottom. They have all these protrusions for attachments of ligaments and muscles. The vertebrae are designed with precise mechanics for flexibility, for example, the neck vertebrae move easier than those in the lumbar area. The spine itself is also designed with a natural curve in three places. This is for shock absorption action as well as for strength and leverage. A straight spine would have no give and not be as strong as a curved spine.

There are seven smaller vertebrae in the neck, the top two called atlas and axis move freely in a twisting, rotating motion and are the only ones without a disc in between them. The common area for disc problems in the neck is at the base (mostly women), at 6th and 7th cervical spine or 1st thoracic spine. However, I seem to find many with stress on the 2nd cervical.

Then we have the twelve thoracic vertebrae in the mid back. These have the ribs attached to them forming the protective cage for the organs. They are less flexible, and the injuries in this area are fewer. The last and largest are the five in the lumbar area of the low back. These are the strongest, yet the most common injuries happen to the lumbar L4-5 and S1 or the fourth, fifth and between the first sacral vertebrae (mostly men). The base of the spine holds some vertebrae that were fused early in life and it's called the sacrum, a common area of injuries as well from straining the back, falls, lifting, or bending over doing heavy work when not properly prepared. Add to this the over use syndrome of putting stress on it for years.

The spine not only has some of the largest muscle groups woven through the vertebrae, but there are also hundreds of small muscles and ligaments that attach to it and provide all types of criss-cross support and movement.

To me, the sacrum and pelvis are the foundation to the whole spinal column as well as the hinge that holds the body together. It's the center of the hips, and there are a tremendous amount of ligaments that attach all of these bones together. Also, some of the larger gluteal muscles attach at this site on the sacrum and these are the workhorses of the body.

The reason for these being such common sites for injuries is that these areas are high stress and gravity points and if there is any misalignment of the body, they take far greater stress or torque. We will look further into the specific areas of the body and joints later in the book.

Although pain may be in the back and or the neck, sometimes it may seem like it's coming from the muscles. Muscles in fact are rarely the cause of this type of pain. Ligaments can be another source of pain and these are considered strains.

There is a medical doctor named John Sarno who actually feels that most back pain is due to muscle and tension. He doesn't believe in irritation or disc injuries causing back pain. In fact, there is another group of doctors that think it's all in our minds. After talking to my surgeon friend Dr. Hiller about that theory he said, "You need to look at the discs and the nerves when you do an operation. Then you see how swollen and irritated the nerves and tissue can be with back pain." So that tells us that the disc out of place either budging ("slipped" is not really accurate) or herniated (torn) does put some pressure on the nerves and eventually the swelling of the nerve causes pain.

With pain comes muscle tension and holding patterns that increase the tension, and thus increase the pressure on the disc, and more disc pressure means more budging or more leakage if it's torn.

This creates a vicious cycle of pain, holding pressure, more pain, etc. It takes great knowledge and experience of what is the primary cause to help a patient in this condition, just as well as what not to do.

One of the reasons for so much controversy about whether back pain is caused from structural problems, discs, nerve irritation, or mental stress is because often in the clinics we see patients with backs that are so out of alignment that we think "how does this person walk around with this back so out of alignment?" Yet some of these have little or no pain or symptoms. Then again, we see another patient with a small vertebra misalignment feeling severe pain. This is giving mixed messages to many doctors. So they often feel that maybe its not structural misalignment that causes pain.

I have seen the worst scoliosis patients, some in severe pain, some in moderate pain, and some with hardly any pain. Scoliosis is a condition where there is a lateral S curve of the spine. You would think these people would be in severe pain all the time. It's because of so many varied symptoms that it's so confusing. There is only one way to deal with this. We have to treat each patient, each condition and injury separately. We cannot lump them all into back pain patients; we need to treat the individual.

I have seen conditions where there is a twist in the spine so severe it causes the ribs on one side to protrude so the person looks like they have a hunchback. On the other hand, you have patients that have gotten the surgery to fix the injured disc and they still have the pain. It's very complex, yet more the reason we need to work together to help all our patients. There are enough hurt people to go around. You never know what is going to help them, or what will work. The key is to do no harm and keep an open mind. The health, the education, and improvement of the patient is what's important.

So if pain becomes our measure, you often don't know what can cause some of these back pains unless you are trained in assessment of the spine. Some have no apparent reason for the pain, it just came on, whereas others are more obvious such as injuries or car accidents. Either way, it takes some knowledge and experience to help these patients, improve and get on the road to recovery.

Most of the experts on the spine are orthopedic and physiatrists, (Physical Medicine) M.D.s, osteopathic (D.O.s), and some chiropractors (D.C.s). Even here we have some controversy. I wish we could just work together for the betterment of the patient and put our differences away. Just as there are many types of back pain and injuries there are many ways to treat these conditions.

Let's start with the mildest form of back pain or tension and work our way to the worst. First of all, everyone on this planet has some sort of muscle tension. This comes from dealing with gravity, lack of muscle tone, too much sitting at computers, or poor posture. Basically, it's from just using your muscles that contract to work. Gravity sucks, and it is a constant stress on the body. If you fight it, you lose, and the result of that is muscle tension, fatigue, and eventually pain.

These muscle tension knots can be a source of pain; usually starting out as discomfort or dull aches. The most common area for modern wo/man is in the neck and shoulders because of stress and sitting for long periods of time in an office. They could also get tight after doing any heavy physical activity.

This muscle tension comes from the contraction of muscles and this stress is accumulative. All our muscles work by contraction, and when continually contracting and not getting stretched or relaxed enough, they tighten up. When the muscle is contracted for an extended period, nutrients in the blood can't get in and toxins from all the cell action can't get out. This forms a chronic stressful and contracted muscle knot. Massage can help break the cycle, but to help it for the long term we need to get to the cause, and that could be just about anything.

The next tension level is muscle spasms, or cramps. These may be more severe knots in your body causing you pain. This pain can create secondary muscle holding patterns, and then you have a whole bunch of muscle tension. Many times these muscle spasms are actually a protective mechanism and secondary to some sort of injury, or structural imbalance. You may have torn or injured a muscle, or just as common, you may have injured a ligament or disc. These conditions can all cause muscle spasms, and although the pain feels like it's in the muscle, it most often is referred pain coming through the nerves from a disc or ligament tear.

The muscles can feel very sore to the touch, and you may have trigger points that are very tender. These are secondary conditions and massage can only help temporarily. Traditional chiropractic care during these acute conditions is also not very effective. The key is determining the extent and source of the injury, give it the appropriate treatment, and if a disc, reduce the impingement of the nerve.

As we see, the muscle spasm is not always the problem unless you are training and have overworked the muscle. The spasm can be a protective mechanism, and these secondary reactions need to be looked at to determine the underlying cause. That is why often just taking pain medication can actually mask the cause as well. And there is an appropriate time for pain medication.

When evaluating an injury, keep in mind that a muscle spasm is a symptom of the injury, not necessarily an injury in itself. Torn muscles of the back or neck area are fairly uncommon unless you are talking about a whiplash from a car accident, or a severe contact sport injury. Vertebrae misalignments, sprained or torn ligaments, and budging or ruptured discs pressing on nerves are the main causes of back or neck pain.

Sometimes we wake up with a pain in the neck, which can sometimes happen from sleeping in a bad position. This is the hardest type of injury to treat with massage. The damage has been happening all night and there may be quite a bit of irritation on the nerve. A doctor can give some anti-inflammatory medication, or just plain aspirin may help. This condition comes from a pinched nerve or stress from a disc in the neck, which can cause pain in the neck or shooting into the shoulder. It will go away in a few days, however, we can aid with massage and sometimes some manipulation.

Of course, that old saying "I just bent over and threw my back out" is usually like the last straw that broke the camel's back. It had been working its way to being out of place or bulging the disc, to the level where it presses on the nerve for quite some time. Then you slept wrong and we have an acute condition that's hard to remedy.

It's not uncommon to have referred pain when you have a pressing disc on a nerve. The nerve may be sending pain messages down the leg or arms depending on where it is. It's a common theory that the further down the pain goes; the more pressure is on the nerve. There are several orthopedic ways to examine the spine to determine the problem. (See the section on the tests for the spine).

When pain is referred though the body it takes a very specific pattern, and the dermatomes give you the map from where it originates. The dermatomes are the areas that allow us to determine which vertebra or nerve is causing the problem. Each nerve exiting out from its specific vertebra has a mapped out area where it sends communication, pain, numbness or tingling.

Injury to the lumbar area often causes pain in the buttocks, or it goes down the leg commonly called "sciatica." In severe circumstances it can reach as far down as the foot or toes, causing numbing or tingling sensations all the way down. Neck injuries can cause pain down to the shoulder, into the arm or all the way down to the hand or fingertips with the same symptoms. Once again, the dermatomes will give you the key to the location at the source. However, if you are not a doctor or working under one, you should be careful to not diagnose this type of injury.

If you have more localized pain it could be that a lower back ligament could be sprained. You need to do the orthopedic tests to determine what it is. With either of these injuries you can feel pain down the leg, across the foot, and ending in the toes. Even some physicians have difficulty determining whether it's a sprained ligament in the spine, or the sacroiliac joint. If you are not familiar with the orthopedic examinations, when in doubt refer to a qualified back and neck doctor.

Weakness in the Muscles of Extremities

We use Kinesiology or the reflex tests sometimes to determine the extent of muscle strength or nerve intervention. Sometimes you feel like you have lost control of your leg or arm during a back or neck injury. The muscles may feel weak or like you have very little control over them. This condition is indicative of a nerve being pinched. I have had patients that could not lift their leg off the table. This could be severe enough that you need to refer them to a doctor. When the nerves are pinched enough to cause this, the motor use is impaired. If this persists, at worst it could cause permanent damage or create a chronic back or neck condition.

The weakness can occur in an arm, hand, leg or foot. It could be accompanied by numbness, tingling sensation, or it might not. Long term neglect of such a condition at worst could also lead to a change in the size and tone of the muscles that are affected. This muscle shrinking is called atrophy. This does not happen too often, as most people get help before it gets that bad. Sometimes the muscle atrophy and weakness is very obvious, but other times it's subtler and can hardly be noticed. To me, this is where prevention therapy comes into effect, by correcting the structure before it becomes a major problem. This is the foundation to my whole therapy and fitness program: Total body/mind alignment. Balance is the key to all things. Structural integration means integrating the structure to make it whole and work together. Operating at the highest level of body mechanics is one of our goals in our massage and exercise program for athletes and patients.

When the injury is in the spine or the neck, that weakness indicates that a bulging or rupture commonly called a slipped or torn disc is pinching a nerve. Sometimes this can be severe enough to interrupt the nerve's ability to communicate with that part of the body. The whole body receives orders from the brain through the nervous system. When a ruptured disc causes intense pressure on the nerve, the electrical impulses can no longer get through. The muscles don't work at their fullest capability, and for athletes this is imperative, because they want to work at the highest level they can. For the rest of us, it's subtler. We may have less energy, feel a little weaker or just not be sure what's going on. A clear example of weakness in a lower back injury is when control of the foot during walking is lost. This is often referred to as "drop foot." The foot drags and flexing the foot is difficult, even walking is a problem with this condition. Of course, it can get really bad, where the person is actually not able to walk at all.

The Tingling or Sensation of Pain

The tingling, like when your arm or leg falls asleep, or that feeling of pins and needles, is an indication of a disc pressing on a nerve, and rarely a muscle spasm. This sensation or tingling, some patients say, feels like hot or cold sensations as well. This can sometimes be a sign of serious neurological trouble. Often, this sensation occurs from some common event, like when you sit too long, or by lying on your arm, and it usually goes away. It can only be serious if it persists. At this time you should consult a doctor.

Osteoporosis

As we all get older we seem to notice how many women are dealing with osteoporosis. It's common in women in their later years, but we believe it starts much sooner than that. The usual traditional medical approach is to prescribe estrogen. This article is not to prescribe or diagnose this condition but merely to educate about integrated medicine (Holistic Approach). Please see your physician for any condition you may have.

Osteoporosis is classified as a disease that creates weakening or thinning of the bones. It's a major problem in our society, and one of the factors in hip fractures and spinal problems such as deformities like "dowager's hump" or in actual spinal compression fractures affecting mostly women in their 60s, 70s or 80s. At this age the body produces less estrogen during menopause. I feel that there are many other factors for the loss of calcium. One is the acid environment we create with our diet; the other may be a deficiency in vitamin D or C, as they regulate the absorption of calcium. Many times calcium in supplements is not even absorbed. The most concentration of elemental calcium, which is the most beneficial of all the types of calcium, is "calcium carbonate."

There are many nutritional treatments available to prevent or improve this condition. It is well known that too much protein in the diet, as well as phosphate containing foods like soft drinks, can contribute to it. Our nation has calcium in everything these days, even orange juice, and it also has the highest concentration in the world of osteoporosis.

Some physicians that work with nutrition are actually saying drinking milk actually does not provide that much calcium to the body. This is rather controversial to all that we have been taught about the benefits of drinking milk. There are other downsides to milk. Casein the protein in milk is linked with many allergies, or if taken too early in life can contribute to immune weakness. Lactose, the sugar in milk contributes to many digestive disruptions if you don't have the enzyme lactase to digest it. Many people are lactose intolerant, so besides all the hormones and antibiotics fed to cows to overproduce milk, it may not be "the perfect food" (Weil). According to Dr. Robert Young this milk sugar is a contributor to creating an acid environment and calcium is then not properly absorbed (see sources).

Most experts agree that nutritional factors play the biggest role. They recommend a diet low in protein, bread and sugar, and high in natural grains, vegetables, and fruit. This diet is alkaline, reducing calcium loss and improving bone growth and repair. It's best to start after the initial growth spurt of most women, which occurs after the late teen years. It seems that small boned women are more prone to osteoporosis than big framed women, and there are ethnic differences as well.

Most Americans have a high intake of acid-promoting foods due to too much protein from meat and dairy products. The body draws bicarbonate, an anti-acid or alkaline chemical, out of the bones to neutralize this acid, and this contributes to the loss of calcium and other minerals. Milk, although high in protein and fat, does not promote an alkaline balance and contrary to most of the advertisement from the dairy industry, does not provide much calcium.

Low blood sugar is another significant factor in women with osteoporosis. Caffeine, alcohol and soft drinks promote calcium loss as well.

Many of us have heard that exercise can help stave off osteoporosis. This is true, however, you don't get osteoporosis and then start to exercise to cure it. Exercise needs to begin early in life. As you exercise you build muscles and you build and strengthen the ligaments and bones as well. It's important to at least walk, as that strengthens the legs, pelvis, and back bones. I believe some mild weight training is even more desirable as it can shape your body. Even older women who start to exercise may benefit and reduce osteoporosis. The body responds to what we call the theory of adaptability, which means the body will get stronger when stressed, whereas the couch potato lifestyle actually does the opposite and contributes to bone loss.

Until recently, estrogen supplementation has been the most common traditional medical approach. Consult your physician (there are pros and cons to estrogen therapy, so be well informed- see caution below. Share this article with your doctor).

A good multi-vitamin and mineral complex
Vitamin A, an anti-oxidant, 30,000 to 40,000 IU for a month, then reduce to 25,000 IU daily
Boron 1-3 mg: Helps retain calcium; stimulates bone formation.
Vitamin B complex with extra B-12, 1000mcg –See physician for injections or use lozenge.
Calcium 1000 to 2000 mg: (the chelated form is best for absorption).
Chromium 300-500 mg: improves insulin efficiency and bone density
Copper 3 mg daily –helps in formation of bone.
Vitamin C 3,000 mg and up daily- anti-oxidant.
Vitamin D 400 IU daily – helps absorbed calcium.
Vitamin E 400 IU daily- anti-oxidant.
Manganese as directed on label –do not take with calcium.
Strontium .5-3 mg – Increases bone density
Silica as directed on label – helps calcium absorption and strengthens bones.
Vitamin K 0.1-0.5 mg – helps calcium crystals join bone's protein matrix.
Zinc 10-30 mg – required for normal bone formation.

Some other products that may be helpful are:

Glucosamine Plus from Foodscience Labs- develops bone and connective tissue.

Bone Builder from Ethical Nutrients , or Bone Defense from KAL Labs, or Bone Support from Synergy Plus. Or Bone Builder with baron from Metagenics

Osteo-B-Plus from Biotics Research Labs

Progesterone: Consult your M.D. Some physicians strongly prefer natural to the standard synthetic progesterone.

Some good sources for vitamins are: Ethical Nutrients, KAL brands, Biotics Labs, Food Science Labs, Freeda Vitamins, Natures Plus, Natures Secret, American Biologics, Now Foods, Nutraceuticals, Source Naturals, Natraen, Marlyn Nutaceuticals, Synergy Plus, Metagenics.

Many calcium supplements are NOT WELL DIGESTED, especially by older people who could lack digestive acid in their stomach. Check your calcium pill by placing it in a small glass of vinegar. If the pill can't dissolve in vinegar in an hour, it probably won't dissolve in your stomach, either (Podell). Check for liquid vitamins (Dr. Robert Young).

Estrogen lowers the risk of bone fractures due to osteoporosis by about 50% when it is taken during the <u>first five years</u> of menopause. Unfortunately, the potential health hazards it poses may not make estrogen the perfect treatment, mainly because it cannot reverse established osteoporosis, nor has it proven very good at preventing menopausal osteoporosis after the first five years.
According to Podell, while estrogen may slow bone breakdown, it does not promote new bone growth or formation. The greatest advantage of exercise, progesterone, and the intense nutritional treatments is that they do seem to stimulate the body to lay down new bone (Podell).

Be sure to check with your physician before undergoing any change in diet or vitamin therapy.

Sources;
Richard Podell, M.D., Andrew Weil M.D., James F. Balch, M.D., Phyllis Balch CNC, and Robert Young, Ph.D.

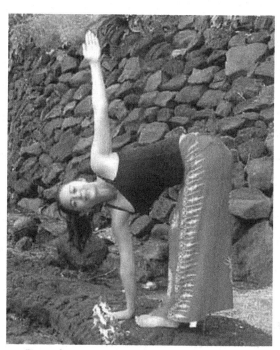

CHAPTER SEVENTEEN
Abnormalities or Diseases of the Spine

Lordosis (sway back)

One of the most common problems of the back we see is the sway back or sagging posture called lordosis. Lordosis refers to an exaggerated forward (anterior) curve of the spine. I believe it's more of a postural problem rather than inherited from our parents. However, there is the possibility that we inherit some of the weakness, and then we copy their postures and habits later in life. (See Feldenkrais, Dychtwald, Rolf.) The body postures follow the mind patterns that we create with our personalities, to a certain extent.

We all have a small anterior curve of the lower spine, a posterior or backwards curve of the thoracic area, and an anterior curve of the neck. There is a purpose for these curves. They are more shock absorbing this way and much stronger for leverage. This is normal and desirable.

I often find that many necks have what they call a reverse curve. That means that it has lost its normal forward curve. It's common to lose this in car accidents or in poor posture. It's only when they get out of balance or exaggerated that they cause problems. In my experience, this leads me to believe that a chronic sway back can lead to ligament stress to the lower spine because it's under constant stress. Also it causes the whole body to compensate, thus increasing the pressure on a specific ligament group or disc. This whole tissue, ligament or disc has double or triple the normal pressure on it. Then all of a sudden, one day you bend down to pick up a newspaper and you are knocked to the floor with pain.

If something in the body or spine structure moves one way, something else has to move the other way. For every action in the body there is a reaction. Many therapists believe that tight psoas muscles cause this sway back condition. Once again, in my opinion, the muscles are not strong enough to pull bones out of place, especially the bones of the pelvis and lower back. They're not strong enough when you consider the strength and density of the bone structure with all those ligament attachments. This condition usually comes from poor habits of improper posture over a long period of time. Of course, it can come from a sudden injury as well, but I doubt it. Treatment must also vary as to the specific situation and person.

Kyphosis (hunchback)

Kyphosis is an exaggerated posterior curve of the spine. This is also common in males more often. It could happen in the mid back region, sometimes called a hunchback, or as a reverse curve in the neck or lumbar area, which are less common. This could be an inherited structural abnormality in its milder form. You see it passed on from parent to child, and it is more common in men.

The potential for weakness can be inherited and then we imitate our parents' habits. Then, it could also be more poor posture and lack of proper exercises that sometimes create this condition. It's not uncommon to have no symptoms other than excessive tension.

However, there are many that have muscle pain and severe tension. It's a posture taken on with the mental connection of carrying a heavy burden, or sometimes males being cave men. Prolonged stress to the back muscles eventually creates more pressure, like a tight string on a bow. Eventually this stress translates to the disc, vertebra, or any joint of the body.

Scoliosis (sideways S curve)

Scoliosis is one of the most common conditions where everyone can see severe misalignment of the spine. It's a congenital condition, usually passed on from mother to daughter. In my experience, more women have scoliosis than men. There are many degrees of scoliosis and depending on the condition, it may not even hurt. Many of us have a mild form of it. It's a condition that makes the spine twist and shift laterally in an S curve.

This causes the muscles in the back to develop differently, some on one side of the spine, some on the other. In extreme cases, it can also cause the ribs to stick out on one side. The shoulders will appear at different heights, as well as the hips. The female patients notice their dresses fit funny. Men may have to take one pants leg up more than the other, and of course, some have so much pain that they have already seen many doctors.

I've treated many patients with scoliosis with different results (15 patients composed of 3 men and 12 women of ages from teens to 60s in one survey of a year). Most patients agreed to 10 session series, which gave me a good base for my study. There are two types of scoliosis. One is called functional scoliosis, which means when you check the patient laying down there is no noticeable curve. However, when they stand up, it's very noticeable. With this condition I have had good to moderate success. Many patients had pain in the back at the worst curve, some patients had pain in the shoulder, as it's in a precarious mechanical position, and others even suffered in the neck. After a series of treatments, more than 85% of these patients had relief of pain. Some actually changed in their postures quite noticeably (six women and one man). Then there were a few others that we couldn't help much (one man, 64, and a woman, 56). I even had two girls with stainless steel rods (ages 16 and 22) placed in their backs because of the scoliosis. Sometimes this is the last resort for this condition. I'm not sure about surgery done for this as most of them still suffered.

I also had a patient with wedge shaped vertebrae. This is structural scoliosis. This condition is impossible to correct, as the vertebrae shape has grown deformed. It's like a wedge and so the body tilts sideways. Then amazingly, the body tilts on the other side of the gravity line and wedges them in the other direction. This type is very rare. I have only seen one patient like this in 30 years. The therapy seemed to help relieve the pain but it would come back if not seen again in two weeks or longer.

I found that through massage and structural corrective exercises, we could reduce the pull of the muscles and give some relief to the patient from the pain. With seven of our patients, their scoliosis totally improved to the point that the before and after x-rays looked like two different bodies. Six others had moderate improvement and 60% less pain. The key was the series of therapy treatments as well as specific, corrective exercises to re-structure the spine through the muscles and ligaments.

Two of the women getting fantastic results were also using the "isolation tanks" before a treatment. You float in saltwater at body temperature inside a tank that is totally dark. It is totally relaxing to the nervous system as you float in the saltwater. It is still a mystery how all this works. Through the seventies and eighties I was fortunate to have three different friends with tanks and did many experiments with this system of meditation. I also felt that the saltwater had a soothing effect on the nerves and brain. Not to mention the deep relaxation throughout the muscles, it is fantastic using this system.

Spondyloisthesis (vertebra off center)

Spondyloisthesis is a disease where one of the vertebrae is pushed anterior or posterior, off the center of the spine. In other words, it's not properly aligned over the vertebrae above and below it. I have seen this condition in the clinic.
It can be a severe enough problem for some patients that it takes some serious therapy to help, especially if there is severe and constant pain. The vertebra could be off by one quarter to one half an inch out of alignment. This misalignment means that people with this condition are more susceptible to pain and injuries in this area, because there is a weak link. This can happen in the lower back, but also in the neck or mid back as well. It is not a very common problem in its severe state, but there are similar problems with less severity.

These are vertebrae out of alignment, too anterior or too posterior or even twisted. Now for the doctors that feel that misaligned vertebrae are not a source of pain, this is the worst condition and demonstrates that theory is sometimes questionable. Just palpate around vertebrae that are out of alignment and you will find pain and tension all around them in all the tissues. The disc itself doesn't really hurt as it has very few nerves or blood flow to it. That's why cartilage injuries take longer to get well because of less blood flow. Plus, if you do not remove the stress, it just can't heal fully.

All of these conditions can create the environment that can lead to a disc injury. The worst condition of a disc injury can cause paralysis. You may not be able to walk or even move when you have this kind of back injury. The symptoms may be different from a specific disc, but in this severe situation, it's unmistakable.

Just lowering your head can cause pain in that area. Sometimes coughing can increase or set off the pain, as well (these are two tests we do to determine if it's a disc). This is because of the connection of the durra matter in the spine that is all connected in the spinal column.

When the disc bulges or when it is ruptured, it can create varying levels of severity and pain. The disc can push and irritate the nerve, or the soft matter flows out and presses on the nerve. As the nerve gets more irritated from the pressure and rubbing on it constantly, it swells and creates more pain. As time continues it gets harder and harder to help this condition with conventional treatments. This is why we recommend that when you first hurt your back, you get medical attention right away. If you have ruptured a disc, the best treatment is using anti-inflammatory drugs. Sometimes a muscle relaxant may be needed or even pain medication. Then rest in bed and let that irritation of the nerve calm down. Even massive amounts of massage and ice can help, but a week in bed can cure this condition. I can attest personally to this, as well as seeing patients in our clinic for years get better if handled immediately.

If you continue to irritate and cause secondary muscle holding patterns, it can last a year or more. You can see patients listing (leaning to one side). When the disc is pushed out to the side, we lean the other direction. Sitting, standing and, of course, walking can continue to put pressure on the nerve and it gets worse and worse. Some people think that "I can't take time off work" and try to push through the pain.

Sometimes we see MRIs that show bulging or torn discs and the patient has very little pain or problems. Wonder why they were there in the first place? Many discs bulge anterior, but because there are no nerves, they are asymptomatic, no pain or symptoms. Eventually, the body re-absorbs the disc matter in the tissue. However, I believe that you have a weak link after that injury, not stronger like in a bone fracture, as I have re-injured the same disc three times in the last fifteen years.

The treatments for a disc injury vary as much as doctors. Having seen hundreds upon hundreds of back patients in a physical therapy clinic during my years as a therapist, I know that this conservative approach works. Sometimes this condition gets better without doing anything but rest. Some therapies may actually aggravate the condition. Therapies involving twisting or adjustments may hurt more than help during the acute state. Massage not performed properly can also aggravate the condition. Medication, traction, trigger point therapy and medical massage properly applied can help. (See the works of Dr. James Cyriax).

Sometimes injections of a steroid with analgesic medicine works quite well to break the cycle. This is called an epidural injection. Then there are some new injections of papain, a papaya enzyme, that help dissolve the disc and get the patient back into recovery. All of this is available from medical doctors that specialize in the backs.

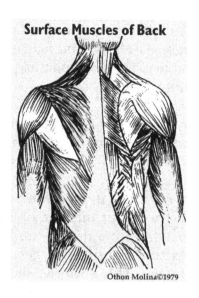

Surface Muscles of Back

Othon Molina©1979

CHAPTER EIGHTEEN
The Thoracic Spine or Mid Back

This area protects the chest cavity and is designed like a cage with the spine and the ribs forming its structure. Consequently, this area has less movement because of that structure. There are fewer injuries to the thoracic area than to the neck and lower back. Often the pain we feel in the upper back is actually coming from the neck.

There are some injuries to this area if you are predisposed to stress and tension. Or you may have some mild scoliosis there, which can tear some of the muscles with a sudden move or from carrying something too heavy. Usually pain in this area, if it is a muscle tear, will hurt with breathing. Sometimes we call it having a rib out. Rib heads don't move too easy unless you have torn some ligaments there or have a weak link. In a car accident you could hurt any area that has unusual tension or scar tissue from an old injury.

You can also hurt this area by lifting something heavy and twisting. You may feel a sharp pain and later it becomes a dull ache. This could last weeks: If you rest for a couple of weeks and it doesn't get better, that's not going to help, seek professional help.

If the rest does not help, it can be treated with manipulation, sometimes just a few treatments help. If you can find the source of the lesion, a muscle tear may be treated with DTF with some success. Then again, medical intervention may be needed in the form of injections. Once again, the treatment used depends on the cause of the pain and the type of injury.

Disc injury to the thoracic area can come on sudden as well as over a period of time. Just like in the neck, we have the same situation of constant poor posture putting stress on certain vertebrae, and we get that tight condition. With lifting or a day of softball at the company picnic, we can cause a disc injury.

Try shoveling snow or gravel for a full day. If you are not used to heavy physical work you can injure a disc this way. Of course, with these conditions of strain you may also have some muscle injuries or intense holding patterns as well. So much depends on how you are living your life. If we realize again that cause and effect; for the sake of this book it just appears this way by our language and in how we approach medicine, we are changing right!

RICE is always good, not the food, even on the deep lumbar areas. Some massage may help, manipulations may help, but traction is not much help in the thoracic area. Then there are the medical treatments like medication or injections. Often it just takes some time for the body to heal itself. After the acute stage we have all sorts of therapies and exercises that can help strengthen the area. Prevention is much better, and less painful.

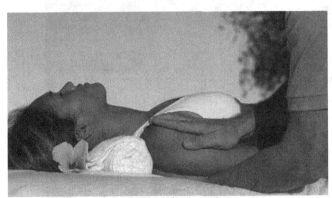

Treatment Massage for the Back

Treatments for injury in the thoracic area vary little from the other areas. The key is to find the source of injury. If it is a muscle, the common ones in the thoracic area are the posterior inter-costals, rhomboids, or sacrospinalis. These muscles weave in and out of the ribs and attach to the vertebrae as well. Sometimes you may injure a rhomboid, other times it may be part of the erectors, these being less common. Either way DTF can aid the body in healing the injury, as well as the use of RICE.

If it's a pesky vertebra out of place it can take your breath away, and if you have a tear in the ligaments it causes such deep pain that you may think you are having a heart attack. Sometimes it's hard to breathe with this condition. The best treatment (if it's going to help) is a series of deep massages and manipulations. There is nothing like a well-placed adjustment to get a vertebra or rib back in place. Of course, if that doesn't work there are always well-placed injections.

We have talked about injections because at times it is necessary to resort to whatever it takes to get better. To me, these, along with surgery, should be a last resort. They should be used properly, at the right time, and with knowledge. I became a believer of using drugs after spending most of my twenty years being against them.

Dr. Portner, in whose clinic I worked in, is a physiatrist, a sports medicine and physical medicine specialist, showed me that there was a place for drugs. With some cases of bursitis, especially of the shoulder, it's the only treatment that is any good. The key is to use them with care, and not just to appease a patient with a chronic condition.

Also, use of injections needs to be followed with the caution to stop training because the tissue can become weakened with steroids and can get injured even worse if the athlete does not stop activity. If steroids are over used, they can cause the tissue to deteriorate and make the problem worse.

Another Molina move for the thoracic spine and neck complex:

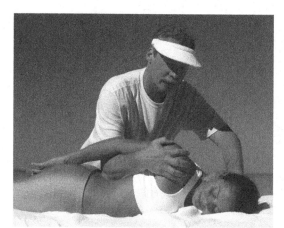 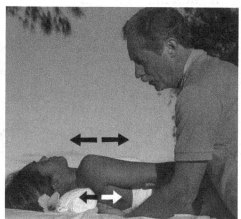

Work the upper thoracic and lower cervical neck. (Left)
Working with the rhomboids muscle and mid thoracic spine (right)

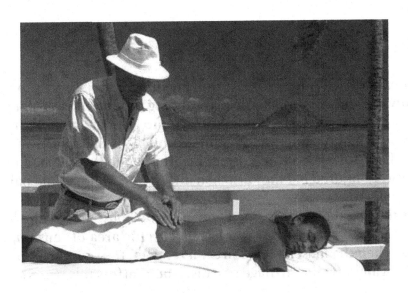

CHAPTER NINETEEN
The Low Back

The mysterious low back, it's a very controversial area of the body. Some doctors think low back pain is totally physical, others, mental. Some say it's due to stress, some say it's because we walk upright. Kind of silly that this back that has taken thousands of years of evolution to develop and it would have any weaknesses. I don't know how it could become such a problem for modern man. What did the cavemen do when their backs gave them trouble, or did they? No one really knows. Also, why do some people have horrible x-rays (misalignments that look like they should be dead) and have no symptoms? Then again, you have someone with a normal looking x-ray with lots of pain. This is the mystery.

Some doctors and therapists like me have dedicated our lives to understanding this mystery. To me, understanding is not important but helping is, and you never know from one individual to another what is going to help. We are all at a loss with some cases and sometimes we have to experiment to see what works. As Dr. Portner said: *"Most back pain gets better responding to time and proper treatment. If treatments are going to be effective, a noticeable improvement should be seen within a few weeks. If no improvement is seen, question whether the treatment is worthwhile and seek alternative treatment. The trick is education; learn to prevent further back problems with correct posture, proper lifting techniques, and correct exercises."*

That emotional or mental stress contributes to pain is just beginning to be understood more fully. The body can create its own cortisone as well as endorphins and histamines that are stronger than anything we make in the laboratory. What causes the body to get out of balance to the point that we have this kind of pain with no noticeable injury? We could ask why forever, and it does not matter why. The key to me is how to best help these people who suffer. We know we need to work together as no one person has all the answers. I have had great success with people who have been given up on by conventional medicine. On the other hand, I have seen people who have been helped by conventional medicine that had given up on natural healing methods. We have the best of both worlds, and if we continue fighting as to who is right, or what the best treatment is, we are missing the point.

Low Back Injuries

The most common low back injury comes from picking up something too heavy. It can also come on gradually through over use, too much bending over on the job, poor posture all your life, falls, etc. You can get a low back injury in an auto accident as well. In fact, I have seen hundreds of auto accident patients and the thing I noticed is that with every individual, even though they may have suffered similar accidents (rear ended), each had not only different areas where they were injured but they also had different symptoms and pain.

The weak link is the one that suffers when you push the body beyond the limits of what you have trained it for or it can handle. If you have a chronic area of tension, you can actually have a weak link. Then the muscle, if it starts there, puts stress on the joint that it works on; the joint, if it has ligaments and cartilage or a disc, then suffers this stress and so on.

We are talking about structural stress, not necessarily mental stress. However, as we said earlier, it could start there and create a weakened or more susceptible condition, too. So often mental stress is cumulative to muscle tension, and along with some physical stress, presto, we have a weak link that is going to suffer.

The commonly referred to "slipped disc" is actually either a bulging disc or a herniated disc (torn). A bulging disc means that it's sticking out of its normal space. A herniated disc means the disc's outer shell has torn, and released the softer material in the middle. This compresses the nerve and can cause pain locally in the buttocks or all the way down the leg. Of course, if you get hit in a football game from the back, it hurts, and you can not only injure ligaments and muscle, but you can also rupture a disc.

Over use can cause muscle holding and injury to the muscle and ligament tissues. If this continues, you bet the disc can be next. I have treated many carpenters for low back problems. For those of you who have built a house, you know how hard this work is. From bending over framing walls, to lifting walls, or carrying heavy timbers or packs of shingles up a ladder, this type of work just wears the body down.

Sacral ligaments sometimes get injured from this intense activity. Take a simple fall on your butt: How many of us have fallen on that gluteus maximus? Everyone. For all the many times we fell as children, we may have appeared to heal quickly, yet it can leave some future weakness that leads to injuries or potential problems for later in life.

This mass of ligaments at the base of the spine that connect the sacrum to the pelvis can create similar shooting pain to that which the disc creates. Muscles very rarely are the problem in low back pain unless it's over use as I mentioned. They go into spasm as a protective mechanism, not as the source of the problem.

Treatment for back injury once again depends on the tissue that is hurt. Muscles and ligaments benefit from DTF if you can reach it. Deep massage is always going to help if done by a professional. Trigger point therapy also helps by releasing the pain and the holding patterns. This seems to help the body heal as well. Traction at some point may work but prevention is always better. Education of how our backs work is important, for all of us are dealing with gravity.

Although it's not always successful for disc injuries, some manipulations seem to help ligament injuries as well as some muscle injuries. Some say by aligning the vertebrae, it takes pressure of the ligaments and muscles, allowing the body to improve. For ligaments, maybe we tear improperly formed scar tissue and it then has the opportunity to heal correctly. However, if after ten or more adjustments you don't get any relief, try something else (Cyriax). That may not be the problem or the solution.

There are several ways to determine if it's a disc injury. First, see a doctor, they will do some tests. Some of the most common ones are these: They will ask if it hurts when you cough. Also, they will have you lower your head, and if both of these are positive, it's very likely they will test your foot or knee reflexes. Sometimes they may have you stand and lean into the area that hurts. This may not be necessary if you are listing (leaning to one side), as this is a very positive symptom of a disc injury.

A disc injury can be very dangerous if it impairs your nerves that help with your bladder or bowel function. This can be serious, so see a doctor right away. This is not too common but it does happen so it's best to be safe. Pain caused in the sex organs can be very serious as well and should be looked at by a doctor.

Of course, I need to mention that for discs in addition to the above treatments carefully applied there are also injections when sometimes a nerve block is needed. An epidural injection is not uncommon to treat severe disc problems. It can also be a test to see if it really is a disc issue. The papain injection is also recommended in severe cases.

I have seen sclorosing (injection of glucose to create scar tissue and stabilize a weak disc or back). Other times it takes traction and the PT (physical therapists) can give you great exercises to improve your back condition. Acupuncture can always help, but if it's structural, it needs to get corrected with a structural treatment. Acupuncture is more for pain control, energy improvement, relaxing the muscles, and increased circulation. Some professionals can use it as a powerful analgesic. Some herbs have even helped disc problems, too. You just never know what is going to work.

The key again is to have an open mind and to realize that whatever it takes to help is what it takes. It could be an Indian medicine man chanting with an eagle feather. I truly believe this, and I have seen it done. I am not making fun of that. I have studied with Indian medicine men and they are holistic. They tap into the unconscious (Spirit) if there is a subconscious (more about that elsewhere). They use bodywork, herbs and rituals to achieve great healing – body, mind, spirit, and nutrition or natural chemistry. We must realize for any healing to happen it's up to us by allowing the healing and by our minds believing in the healing. Some say it's the subconscious, but why can't it just be the mind, period. Why break it all up?

Surgery should always be the last recourse. Using drugs can be great for treating pain patients, but always with great care with that and with injections I have seen many patients get better. It takes all kinds of medicine these days to help some people. Even my surgeon friends say the same thing. They are very conscientious these days. There are plenty of people that really need surgery. Most doctors are very conservative, and that means concerned. They try everything else first. You can't be in this profession and not care. They do surgery when it's needed as the last resort. Before it gets to that point though, we work conservatively, looking at each condition specifically, and treating the patient with all the tools available to us naturally!

There is a new procedure for the severe disc injuries called IDET. What they do is insert a wire into the spine with a little camera, as they do with arthroscopy knee surgery. The wire is heated and cauterizes the disc, causing it to close up. This is a new procedure and there are only a handful of doctors that do this. It's less invasive than conventional surgery that fuses your spine because, unfortunately, even then you never know if the problem will be corrected. This is another aspect of how we don't understand back problems: You would think once you fix it, the pain goes away. Well, that is the mystery of the spine. As I said before, some doctors think it's all in our mind. Well, of course, it is – everything is in our mind. We can still help and treat the symptoms until the patient does the mind work and understands what the body is trying to say with the pain.

This is very important information for anyone with back problems!

If you hurt your back it is usually a disc problem and if you take care of it right away you will be able to heal it faster. I have used this approach with hundreds of patients as well as with my other colleagues. It seems to be the best approach:

1st See a doctor that specializes in backs. Stay in bed, don't sit or stand or even walk much. Most importantly, don't do any exercises that flex the spine (bend forward). The most important exercise to do is to arch the spine, as in the cobra (lying on the ground like you are going to do a push-up, keeping the pelvis flat on the ground and keeping the butt muscles relaxed (see exercise below).

2nd The doctor who is experienced in treating backs will prescribe some anti-inflammatory drugs. Depending on the severity of your condition he may even recommend some muscle relaxers or pain pills. These medications during the early stages are great and can greatly increase the healing. Even using a back brace during this early time is especially beneficial particularly if you are listing (leaning to one side).

3rd Use ice every day, all day if the pain is severe. Doing the cobra while icing it will help pull the disc in. If the full cobra is too much, do the second exercise or what we call the sphinx by just rising up on your elbows. These exercises are the best. An alternative is the cat-dog but make sure you don't go into flexion.

4th Consult with a professional that can guide you to healing the condition. Many times medical doctors don't have the training, and you need to get therapy. Sometimes traction helps with medical massage, and at the right time chiropractic can help, although I have seen it cause hurt during the acute stages. Most important is the alignment of the hips and spine; for the long term recovery this is imperative. The corrective exercises I give are mostly common to physical therapy. I have also developed some of my own that will help take the pressure off the disc. Think about it: If your pelvis is twisted or higher on one side than the other, there will still be pressure on the disc. I believe that for a disc to be injured it has suffered this pressure for a long time, as discs are part of a very strong system. Muscle tension is the way the body compensates for this misalignment and with that it compresses the spine thus breaking down the disc over a period of time. So sometimes with the right conditions such as tension, stress, too much work, just by bending over one day or twisting while carrying something, it can force that weak disc out of place. With either a bulge or an actually torn disc (herniated) you need to work intensely to get it back to health.

Let's review what some of the tools are that professionals may use for disc problems, besides the drugs, which I think are very beneficial if you get them right away. Later on they are less effective, in fact, everything is less effective if you wait a week or more to get help. Go see your doctor right away if you hurt your back, don't wait! Rest in bed is the best and most important therapy you can do along with the medication. Obviously your body is talking to you very loudly, so pay attention, take some time to reflect on you life and listen to your body. Don't walk around and don't sit. Lie down and do the extension exercises with ice. This is not only critical in the early stages, but it will also help all the way through.

Deep massage with an alignment technique is great. The key is to take to pressure off the disc. The problem with deep massage without attention to alignment or with too much twisting is that it can actually make it worse. When you relax the muscles that are holding, it may put more pressure on the disc at least temporarily. Rolfing has a good technique for lengthening the torso fascia. Trigger point therapy can ease the pain and relieve the muscle tension. Chiropractic during the acute phases has mixed reviews, depending on the chiropractor. Gentle work seems to be more effective, but at other times it's just too painful for some patients. It is definitely helpful after the acute phase for alignment. Sorry, chiropractors, but I have found this to be true. Two of my best friends are chiropractors and I use them myself, but as I've said many times, it depends on the patient as well as the doctor. During the later stages after the swelling has gone down may be the time for chiropractic as well as physical therapy or traction. That seems to be the time when it is most effective. Acupuncture will not correct structural problems, but it can help with the pain or even swelling. However, I work directly with many of the best acupuncturists, and they refer their patients to me when there is a disc problem for body alignment.

5th. Once you have injured a disc you have a weakened area for some time. Remember, this tissue heals very slowly. It takes many years sometimes to totally heal a ligament if it came from improper posture, which I think is the most common reason, from slouching all your life or from too much sitting and no exercise. You need to start to change your posture and habits. Yoga, Pilates, Alexander, Feldenkrais or Aston Patterning are many techniques that can help with that. You need to strengthen the abdominal muscles because most often this is a big problem area especially if you are a male and have a large stomach. By the way, most back problems are associated with males.

Since posture is one of the biggest problems with the back, doing the right exercises is critical for improvement. Some of the exercises that are recommended are counterproductive, such as bending over to touch your toes! Never do that, unless you have been shown the right way to do it. Anyway, you can get the same stretch if you sit on the ground and touch your toes without the pressure on your spine. Most flexion exercises are not great for us. These are when you bow your back backwards. It's best to keep the spine flat at the low back for certain stretches. There are even some Pilates moves that I would be very careful with, especially if you have had a back problem. Get some expert advice and always remember to consult with your doctor before starting an exercise program.

6th. Here are some of the most common tests for disc problems:
  a. Does it hurt your back to lower your head?
  b. Does it hurt if you cough?
  c. Can you bend over without pain?
  d. Can you arch your back without pain? Usually if these four cause problems, it's a disc.
  e. There may be a need for more leaning into the pain if it's on one side or the other. This will often reproduce the pain, or cause a shooting sensation down the foot.
  f. Lastly, we may twist and find out if this pain is made worse by doing that. Note that these tests should be done by a doctor and care should be taken in doing them.
  g. There are other obvious signs such as listing (leaning to one side), which is a common disc reaction. The body is trying to take pressure off the disc.
  h. Shooting pain or numbness down the leg or into the buttocks is another sign.
  i. Of course, if you can't even walk or sit, you know what you have.

See your doctor. You can do the first two tests yourself with no problem and if you have the last two symptoms, well, we are pretty sure you have injured a disc. Take care of it immediately and get into bed as soon as possible. I have seen people get better right away, but if not taken care of properly, it can last for years. Believe me, as I have personally had the experience as well. If you have a back problem, get my next book, *The Better Back Book.*

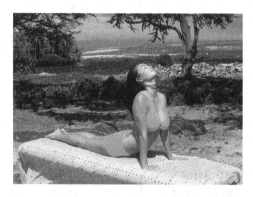 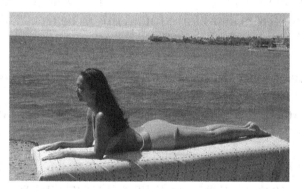

The cobra (left), or extension of the spine. If this is difficult don't push it do the alternate pose the sphinx (right). Both of these are some of the best and easiest exercises to do when your back is hurting. They are the best for assisting the disc to return back to it's normal place and help reduce the tension. Also quite effective for the back muscles as well.

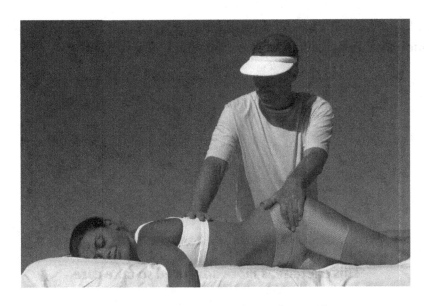

A Nice Way To Lengthen The Back:

Slowly lift patient from their anterior iliac spine, not grabbing hard, and gently pull up the hip while pushing on your side of the spine with your palm. Start at the low lumbar and work your way up each vertebra at a time, drop the hip every vertebra and lift again as you go. If you find tight and resistive muscles, gently massage and friction them as well this will help. Use deep breathing and pull up as they exhale.

With all the troubles that modern people or we earthlings have had with the back, I find it imperative to just take the time and take care of your own. No one can do it ALL for you. It just takes knowing something about the body and just rolling up your pants and diving in. The best strategy I know about everything I have tried is to start out gently, even if you are a big, strong bodybuilder. Most bodies I have encountered in my career are out of alignment; the least were two of the top Olympic athletes of the late seventies.

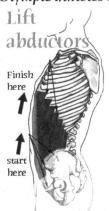

Lift abductors

Finish here

start here

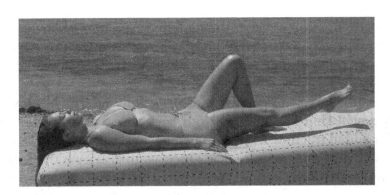

The Abdominal Lift; just sitting and contracting your abs as you lift the torso (left). This takes pressure off the discs. This is also good for when you are doing any exercise as it allows you support and initiates all other movement from the core.

Right; another important exercise to start building your core muscles. Lifting one leg at a time, keeping one on the ground is for beginners option below more advanced.

The object is to keep your abdominal muscles contracted and move the legs back and forth (top one at a time) bottom two at a time bicycling back and forth.

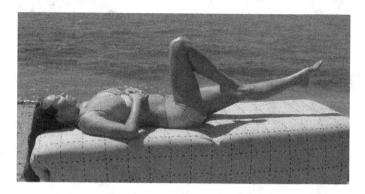

This exercise is more advanced so take care.

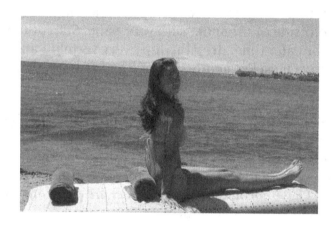

Lengthen Your Own Low Back

Home made traction to assist the body in reversing the stress of gravity throughout the day, the is a great way to get your body relaxed as once the curves are in the right place the muscles can relax instead of holding us in our tension pose.

Starting with two towels one for your neck and one for your low back.
Just lay down! That will lengthen your back. Use a towel under your low back and under your neck for added traction. This is homemade traction at its best, easy to do and takes very little skill, it will do wonders, just try it. Once again gravity is the force we all are subject to, and it exerts its force on our bodies. If we fight it we loose and it becomes stress and tension.

My philosophy is simple, do as many exercises we can that reverse the pull gravity has on our bodies. Hanging up side down has been around since the seventies; we did that after tree planting all day. You can only stay upside down for so long, without training even dangerous so just be careful with all exercises in general. These are beautiful because they are the easiest to do, don't get me wrong just cause they are easy, they are very powerful if done regularly, regularly, that is the key.

I start all the moves to loosen the spine on the ground. I just think it may be less stressful on any back. Most twisting is not usually recommended if you have a strained back or some old ligament injury. You could even push out your own disc. The key is to go easy with anybody when you start any exercise program, (yes, the commercial) and always consult with your doctors.

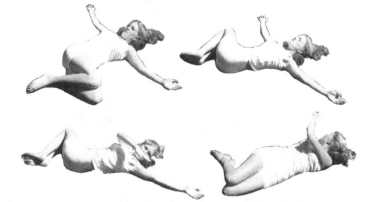

Lengthen the spine gently with knees bent, and then open.

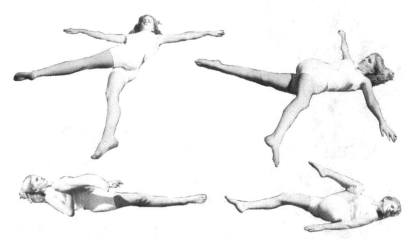

• The top two ways to lengthen the spine are done by very gently lying on the ground.
• The bottom two moves are great, and the key is to keep your spine in neutral and suck up those abdominals. These are general stretches, using the theory of mirror or stretching for your particular alignment (See my other exercises) can be more effective.

At the same time that you are holding the abs like a good corset, you lighten them so that you take all the pounds of stress off the spine and discs. You see, at the same time you are strengthening all the core muscles and all the abdominals and deeper structures. That's also the basis of yoga and Pilates, Alexander, Aston, etc.

I recommend more extension of the spine and hardly ever flexion. Yoga, of course, is the greatest when and if they use the knowledge of Kinesiology or understand body mechanics, those few that may have some potential low back problem. I have even seen Pilates, which I believe, is one of the best all around programs in addition with most yoga, Hastanga, or whatever name you want to call it. God, it's thousands of years old, you would think we could learn something from that. However, don't get stuck in just being an ancient monk. Use technology as well and you have new alchemy, Geometrics.

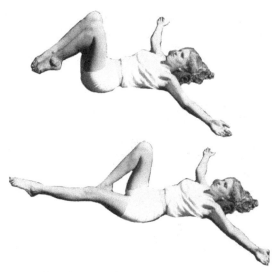

These two are partial strengthening and when done side to side, they lengthen as well.

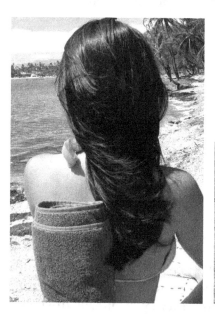

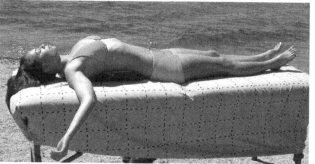

Another great one especially if your shoulders really are tight and pulled forward, or you have large breasts and get stressed or if your head is too far forward and you have a hump. Place towel vertical on your spine ending below your last thoracic vertebrae (Left) then lay on it, it will stretch your pectoral muscles as well as take the stress off your upper back lower neck. Only a few minutes at a time will all my exercises until you build up for at least five to ten minutes.

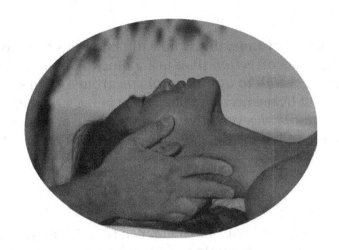

CHAPTER TWENTY
The Neck

The neck and its functions are very important, which is why I always start my therapy there. If the neck is blocked and out of alignment, in a way it cuts the brain off from the rest of the body. It still could be a secondary problem area, nonetheless, necks are very important.

The neck muscles are for stabilizing the head and movement. They are not for holding the head up. Remember, if you are doing that, gravity will win. When we are properly aligned, the bones are designed to hold us up with very little muscle action. That goes for the whole body as well as the neck. The head weighs from ten to fifteen pounds depending on your size. The muscles of the neck at the front (anterior), or flexors, are weaker than at the posterior side, the extensors. They weigh less than a few ounces all together. If they have to hold your head up all day, they fatigue. Then you have all types of compensation through tension. The tight muscles and the tension can even contribute to that headache after work.

Turning the neck involves the muscles at the side such as the sternocleidomastoid, and others working together. There are usually several muscle groups working together to make a movement, as well as their antagonists (muscles that work against or stabilize).

Neck Injuries

The most common neck injury, apart from waking up with a stiff neck, is a strain of the neck muscles. This could be from a minor tear of a muscle tissue to an actual sprain of a ligament. This can be caused by many factors; any sudden motion can injure predisposed tense areas. Take, for instance, that you have a stressful job, and you sit all day at a desk, which includes about half of the population. Then you're invited to play a nice friendly game of softball at the company picnic. At some point you turn your head too hard and further than your muscles were prepared for, and wham! You've hurt your neck.

Another common injury to the neck, of course, are auto accidents, and there could also be severe injury to the muscles, ligaments, as well as the disc.

The muscle spasms that come from all these type of injuries are secondary, protective reactions. Working on them may help, however, as in all healing you have to get to the cause.

If it's happened over a period of time, this is how the body gets to a susceptible condition. Then it takes more long term correction than just a quick manipulation. However, even a manipulation sometimes can work to turn the problem around. You still need to determine the cause. Torn muscles and ligaments don't like either being stretched further or the quick movements of a manipulation. However, misaligned vertebrae or discs that could be relieved by a manipulation respond well in the right circumstances. You just need to know what tools to use and when.

Test for Neck Injuries

Ask all the right questions and find out what happened first. When you have some clue as to how they hurt themselves, start with gentle tests. Passive movements first: have the patient look to one side, then the other and notice pain or limitation in the movement. If it hurts with the motion, it could be a ligamentous injury or muscle. Full flexion of the neck, pain looking down, could be a ligament as well. Then, complete extension (looking up) - pain in extension could be a disc.

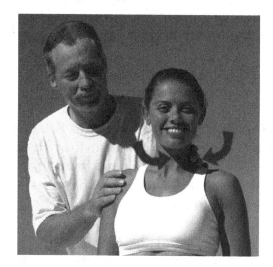

Simple, easy test: Look both directions, note which way there may be pain, then have them look up, extension, and down, flexion. Pain in extension can often be a disc. (See further)

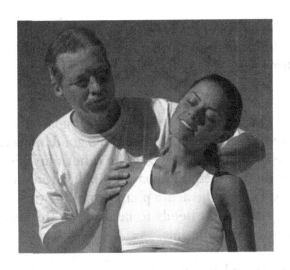

Then check for disc injury, first taking it to the side gently.
Then flexion and extension.

If these don't hurt then we start with resistive movements to determine if it's a muscle injury. See specific muscle tests for further detail.

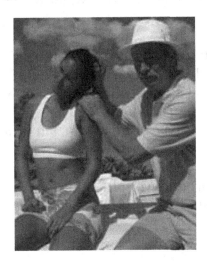

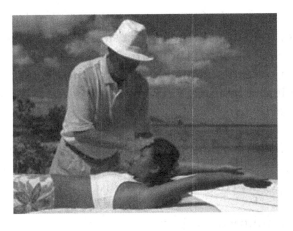

For muscles suspected of injury, test the muscle in a partial contraction and resist the action of said muscle, Upper trapezius shown here.

Anterior neck flexors being tested for neck injury. The muscles should be done after all the easy testing is done first.

Last, if there is limited motion in one direction as you move it, it may cause the pain or referred pain, and then it once again it could be a disc. The final test would be to compress the neck into the side that you feel has the protruding disc. This too will duplicate the pain or the sensation they are feeling.

Treatment for ligament or muscle tear

For any injury involving muscle or ligament, we use RICE (Rest Ice Compression and Elevation). Since it's in the neck, elevation is relative. I would lay them down, as long as their head is above the heart. The treatment is DTF (deep transverse friction massage). Be careful to apply at the patient's tolerance level of pain. DTF can aid in the healing of strained muscles and ligaments; however, great care must be taken when working on the neck with ice.

Traction, if it were a ligament or muscle, would not be a good idea at this point just as deep longitudinal massage on the lesion would also not be a good approach. Why stretch an over-stretched or pulled muscle or tissue? Massaging the other muscles in the holding pattern or that are compensating for the pain would always help, but remember, we need to get to the cause to get the best results. During the acute phase is not the time to do structural alignment or traction to increase mobility. That needs to be done in the second phase of treatments. We want to work on reducing the symptoms.

Diathermy (electronic heat) and ultrasound (sound waves that create heat) have some significant use in this situation because they increase the blood flow that helps the body to heal. I prefer ice during the acute stage for at least four or five days. Use of ice in the neck requires some patience and experience. The DTF with the ice cube is my preferred method. These are common traditional treatments. Even acupuncture helps during this stage to accelerate healing and reduce swelling. This could be a borderline situation where medicines or seeing a doctor is advisable.

The next level of severity with this kind of injury may require seeing a doctor for medicines or an injection. Sometimes a steroid injection into a muscle or swollen area can help break the cycle of pain. There are also proliferant injections, sometimes called sclorosing (when done on the spine) that help create scar tissue on ligaments to help bind the tear and accelerate healing. Very few doctors are skilled in or use this type of treatment, but it can be very effective.

Traction or manipulations at this stage are not very productive, although I have seen improvement at the later stages with these therapies. Most of the time in the clinic we were always very conservative with disc injuries.

A disc injury to the neck

Injuring a disc in the neck hurts severely, and sometimes no matter what you do it all hurts. Just holding the head up can be difficult. Of course, this type of injury can happen just as easily with a sudden twist in sports or from a car accident as it can from developing over a period of years. We don't really know what causes this type of injury because of so many varied reasons. We can only guess that improper posture is a possible cause and that over a period of time we have put unusual stress and pressure on certain discs. Because the ligaments are stressed by misalignments, they can exert more pressure on the whole structure until one day the disc presses on the nerve severely enough to cause the pain. When this happens it can come on with just the turn of the head or even sleeping in the wrong position. Often this pain shoots down the shoulder, or into the arm or hand. This is the same kind of circumstance that happens when somebody bends over, and "throws their back out." Or, they can just turn their head and "throw their neck out."

The tests above show us if it's a disc or a ligament, however, if you're not experienced in these methods of diagnosis, it's easy to get confused, so always consult with a doctor if you have any doubt.

Treatment for disc injuries

There is very little most people can do for these types of injuries, unless they are informed. RICE helps, and resting may do more than you would think. By rest, we mean lying down for a few days. Taking aspirin reduces the inflammation, which can also help (according to most doctors). First you can avoid the positions that hurt, and minimize the motion. Then there's a neck brace: It's a great tool to assist the body in holding the head with less effort. Much like using a back brace, it takes some pressure off the disc. These devices are normally available through doctors. Other medical treatments are injections; they are tricky but can be done, as well as manipulations. You have to be extremely well-trained and be very careful. The wrong move or an injection not well-placed can hurt the patient even worse, or not help at all. We are not always sure why low force manipulations work at this stage sometimes, and at other times they don't work at all. Trigger point therapy relieves the pain, and so does working on the muscles that are involved. The key is to not make it worse. Some traction may help during the second level of treatment as well as corrective exercises. In my experience, it's not that effective as it is during the acute stages.

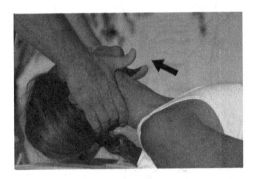

Gentle neck traction, later in the second phase of treatments, can be very beneficial. In fact, I use it as a regular treatment. Since gravity is constantly pulling down on our necks, traction is a great part of all my treatments. We stretch you to new patterns in my work, as well as doing deep tissue massage and movement enhancement.

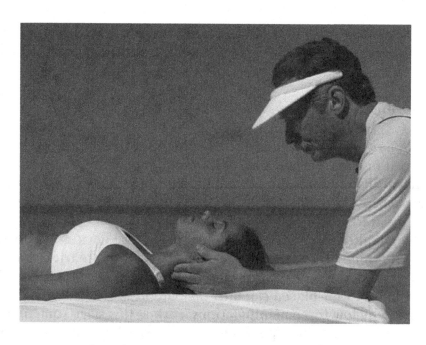

CHAPTER TWENTY ONE
Muscles of the Neck

Levator Scapulae

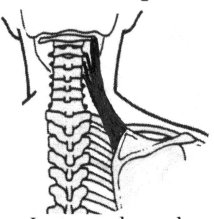

Levator scapulae muscle

Origin: Transverse process of the upper four cervical vertebrae.

Insertion: Medial superior border of the scapula above the base of the spinous border of the spine of the scapula.

Action: Elevates the medial margin of the scapula as in shrugging the shoulder up to the ears. It's a third class lever. Helps in bending the neck to one side.

Palpation: It's difficult to feel the whole muscle because it's under the trapezius. However the insertion is very much palpated, as it's a very tight and stressed in most people.

Strengthen: By doing shoulder shrugs with dumbbells in hands. It acts in conjunction with the upper trapezius muscle.

Lengthen: By bending the head off to one side, you can get a good stretch on the opposite side from where the head is going. You can also flex the neck forward and at a slight angle to get another stretch on the muscle.

Massage: Massage of the neck and shoulders works very specifically on this muscle. With the long strokes on the neck (patient supine), moving upwards. As well as downward strokes with the hands pushing inferior, giving a stretch to levator and trapezius as you push. Also, with patient prone we do some deep longitudinal massage starting at the medial superior border of the scapula up to the base of the scull. Cross fiber work is also very effective on this muscle and we work the origin as well as the insertion. Sometimes I stretch the neck to get some length on the muscle and then cross fiber with my thumbs while the patient is supine.

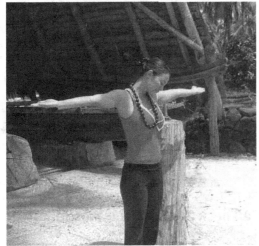 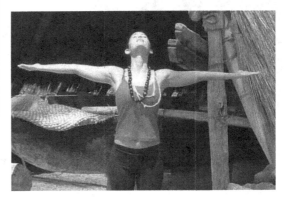

Neck stretch, never do full rotations, to stretch your neck start with rolling the neck in the front (Left) with half circles then do the back (right).

Splenius muscle

Origin: The lower half of the ligamentum nuchae and the spinous processes of the seventh cervical and the upper five thoracic vertebrae.

Insertion: Transverse processes of the upper four cervical vertebrae and the base of the skull toward the mastoid process (near the erectors).

Action: Extension of the head and neck pulling on one side brings neck to the side contracting. It also twists the head to the right with right contraction and to the left with left contraction.

Strengthen: It's a very important group to work with for the extension of the spine. In football it's doing bridges with the head on the ground, or pulleys with straps on the head. There has to be resistance. One other way is while lying prone, you interlace the hands behind your neck and do extensions using the erectors, and the resistance on the neck will work this and the levators as well as the upper erector group.

Lateral stretches for the neck are great to lengthen the muscles take it easy and watch yourself if you can in a mirror so that you stretch even. Make sure to do both sides

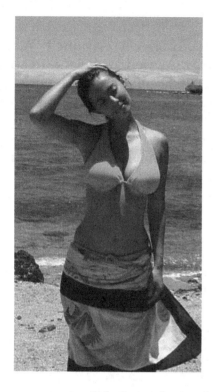 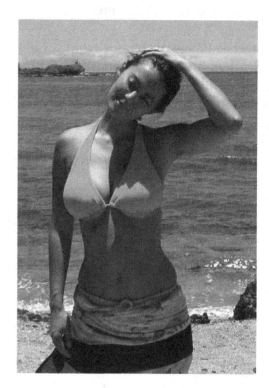

Straight lateral stretch for the over- all neck and trapezius muscle.

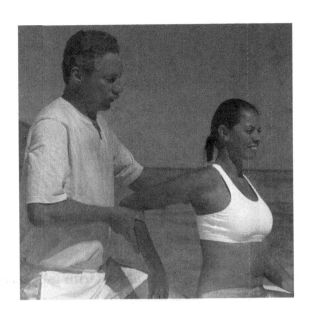

CHAPTER TWENTY TWO
The Shoulder

The shoulder is one of the areas most difficult to treat. Think of the motion of the shoulder. It has the largest range of motion of any joint in the body. What that means is that it's a very complex working mechanism. Because the shoulder needs to have such extreme range, it does not have many ligaments structures holding it in place. There are mostly muscles tied in from the back of the scapula, the shoulder, and arm, as well as the pectoralis groups, the deltoids. . . need I go on. There are lots of muscles holding that shoulder together.

The bones that make up the shoulder are the humerus, the clavicle, and the scapula, which holds the shoulder's ball and socket joint. This is another big reason why it has such a wide circle of action. This is where most of the injuries to the shoulder happen. Most pain, oddly enough, is felt in the middle of the deltoid at the proximal end of humerus.

If we are to help with any part of the body we must know how it works, why it works, and what could it possibly be when it doesn't work. Sound confusing? That it is when it comes to the shoulder.

The shoulder is one of the hardest areas of the body to help by the use of massage. Let's look at the different ways we get shoulder problems. The most common is bursitis, or an irritated shoulder. This can result from an injury where you damage the bursa, the sack that holds the fluids in the shoulder joint to keep it lubricated. Falling on your hand or landing on your shoulder (football) can create a pain and swelling in this joint. It starts to make most wide arm movements painful.

It could also come from long, slow, improper mechanical action on it. The over use syndrome can happen on any part of the body, since when you are not mechanically sound you will stress the joint. Palpate the front aspect of the shoulder (see picture following)

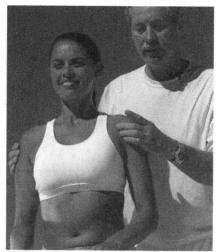

Palpate for tenderness on anterior, superior, and posterior aspects of the humerus and its attachments.

Testing the shoulder is a regular body treatment for me, mainly because it's a common source of stress especially if the shoulders are rounded, and there is some pectoralis muscle tension. You can just check the insertion of the pectoralis, as well as the origin of the biceps to find there is a lot of stress on these tendons.

Much of shoulder pain can be referred pain, coming from the neck or upper thoracic vertebrae. The other common pain is overuse as we said, but that is tendon tension and tendonitis at the farthest onset. Pain in this area can be very diffused throughout the shoulder and upper arm. This is the difficulty, as it is on the C-5 dermatome, so we have to be specific in our tests to find out what the problem is.

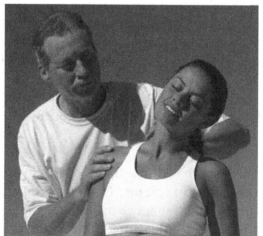

Test for the neck to rule out referred pain.

After that, do extension under control and check for any referred pain down the arm or into the hands.

If movement of the neck causes the shoulder pain, then check the neck further.

The Test for Bursitis (Inflamed Shoulder Joint)

Testing for bursitis, or limited range of any joint or muscle group, will give us an evaluation of the mechanics working on any joint. Imbalances here cause intense stress on any system. Passive abduction may create the worst pain. You will find external rotation is less painful. If you palpate the shoulder you can find scar tissue or knots in the sub deltoid bursa.

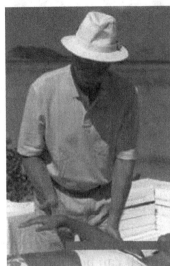
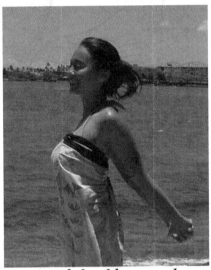

Testing the subscapularis muscle   good shoulder stretch

Check for full rotation of shoulder in both directions.

The Subscapularis Tendon

A common shoulder injury is tennis, pitcher's or swimmer's shoulder. This is when you have injured the subscapularis tendon. The test is to have the patient supine with arm in a 90 degree and push posterior and the therapist resists with anterior pull. It's in this action that the pain occurs. The problem so many athletes as well as other people have is that we create little tears every time with a small injury. Then that creates scar tissue. This is in an area hard to reach with DTF. So you play tennis or softball real hard at the company picnic and you hurt for a week or two. Often times a month is not uncommon, and the wonderful body heals again. So we start to feel better. That scar tissue is brittle and we create a potential injury site again. RICE will always help any injury, but ultimately it make take some medical intervention.

Supraspinatus

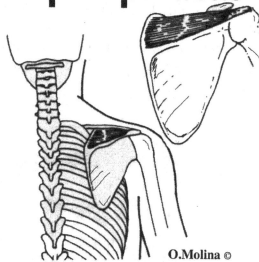

O.Molina ©

The Supraspinatus

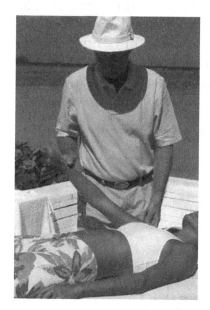

The Supraspinatus Test

There is a different shoulder injury if it hurts to lift your arm on the top of the shoulder. This muscle helps lift the arm before other muscles come into play. It can be injured with falls, or by trying to lift or push harder than it is built for. Take the arm out (Abduct) at about a 30 or 40 degrees angle and push in (medially) as the patient tries to push out (laterally) with a straight arm. The pain will be usually near the tendon. (Insertion)

Infraspinatus

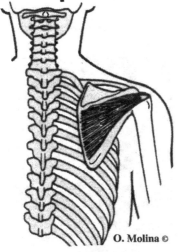

Infraspinatus

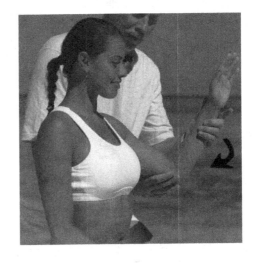

Test

The back side of the shoulder is the location for the infraspinatus, used in hitting a backhand tennis stroke, playing baseball, or football. This pain is usually felt in the back of the shoulder. The muscle originates in the medial edge of the scapula, and inserts at the posterior aspect of the humerus. This muscle can be rather weak, mainly because we do more internal rotation of the shoulder than external rotation. In weight training, they do more pectoralis work than working on those very specific muscles.

Test

Have the person with their arm in a 90% angle, place your hand on their wrist and resist their external rotation or backhand. This will hurt the muscle more if it is the problem.

Biceps Brachii

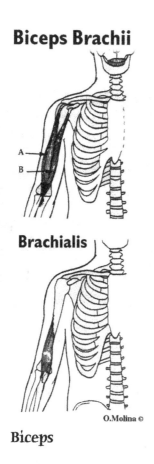

Biceps

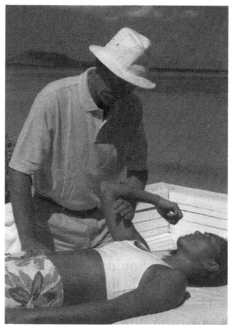

The general biceps test.

The biceps are actually two muscles that insert at the elbow joint. These muscles don't get injured too often but can also cause pain in the shoulder that we should rule out. It could, of course, be injured down at the elbow, but that is less common. Trying to lift something heavy, usually weight training, hurts this muscle.

The test for the biceps is to have the person with their arm bent palm upwards. Put your hand on the wrist and have them try to curl their arm. You resist and notice the area that may have the pain. Go slowly always on all tests. In fact, if there is pain without resistance, have them first move the muscle you suspect and then contract the muscle 50%. Then if still in doubt, up to 75% of a contraction with resistance.

Triceps

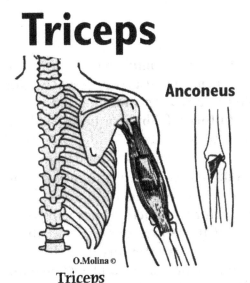

Anconeus

Triceps

O.Molina ©

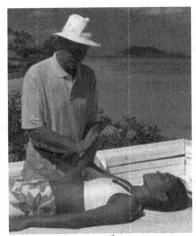

The test

There is another muscle injury to the upper arm and shoulder area, the triceps. It's even less common than the biceps; it is three origins at the posterior part of the humerus, and turns into a large tendon at its insertion into the elbow. Pushing yourself up with your arm will cause pain.

The biceps test:

To test the biceps, have the person supine or sitting, and have their elbow and arm at a 90%. Have them turn palms down, and push inferior to their feet. You resist that action by holding the wrist with an open palm. Pain will be felt at the back of the shoulder and somewhat inferior.

Treatment for all these tendonitis conditions is the same: RICE, and DTF will always help any tendon injury improve if you can get at it. However, the difficulty is doing it correctly so that you don't cause more irritation. The more acute the condition, the softer you work, and more icing need to be done. The more chronic condition, then you can go without ice and do deeper work to break up the adhesions.

Massage is great for these conditions, since you increase the circulation as well as reduce some of the peripheral muscle tension and possible injuries. Any time we can increase circulation to a soft tissue tear, the healing time is quicker.

One shoulder pain that we can't help much with massage, and manipulations can actually make it worse, is the bursitis of the shoulder, acute or chronic. The shoulder pain most people have that comes on gradually or just appears out of the blue is bursitis (see aboveo. When you have pain after sleeping on this shoulder, it's often bursitis.
Shoulders are tricky, so have them see a doctor if you have any doubts. This is the one that definitely needs a doctor's help, as one of the best treatments is to inject it with corticosteroid medicine. It will reduce the inflammation within a few days to a week. It's important to rest it and not strain, as you may get a worse injury. The medication can actually weaken that tissue as it reduces the inflammation.

The next part of the shoulder: the ligaments.

Where the acromion process and the clavicle meet is the acromioclavicular joint. An injury to this area does not cause pain to run down the arm; it's at a very precise point in the anterior, superior part of the shoulder. It is called a separated shoulder and is common in sports. It can also happen by falling down hard, or falling off a bike or horse, and landing on an outstretched arm. There are two ways to put stress on the joint to see if it's those ligaments. Palpation is great for finding this injury. Massage does not do much, although DTF applied with ice and in the acute time could reduce the recuperation time. These injuries if left alone will take a few months to heal. They could be re-injured and then they could last half a year. If you suspect a serious tear, refer to a doctor. They will take an x-ray with the patient holding something heavy and see if there is a separation of the shoulder joint. Once again, injections are some of the best treatments for this condition, corticosteroid, or a proliferant as it can help build up the new tissue and get you pain free.

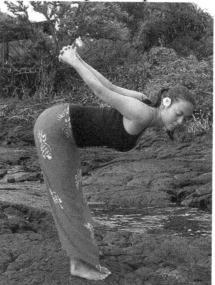

A good stretch and strengthen exercise for the shoulder, note low back is flat no flexion; this is also lengthening the hamstrings and back muscles.

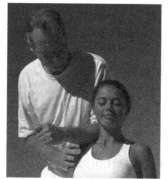 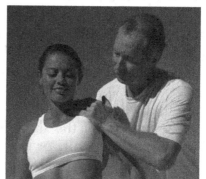

A cool move to loosen the shoulder; first iron out the traps for a few minutes (left). Then take the shoulder and mobilize it all around the sockets and muscles relax. (Right) Following is a series of moves that I do for the shoulder.

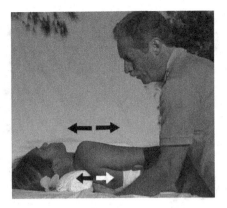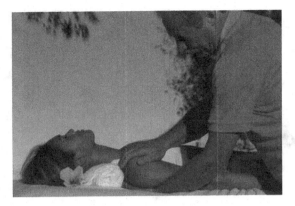

First reach underneath the shoulder and put fingertips on the Rhomboids. Pull and push the arm and create a saw action with shoulder and arm pressing into the muscles. Keep working front and back simultaneously.

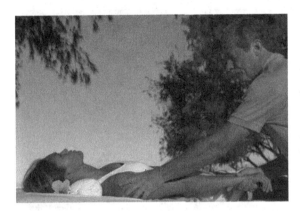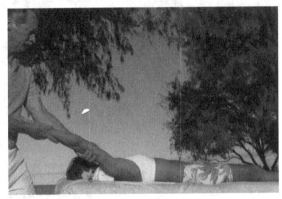

Then lengthen the arm inferior opening the socket. Follow laterally around to the top of the body and lengthen the arm overhead (be careful with these moves if they have shoulder problems.

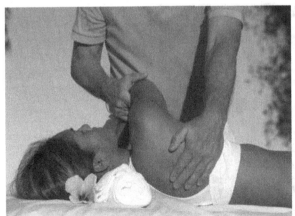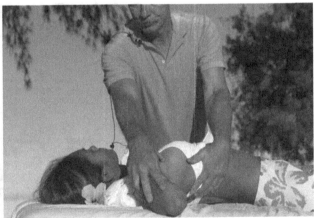

After that movement now take them by the arm and stretch the back and shoulder with one move, use your body weight and not your muscles (left). Then take it back the other way supporting their arm, move back across the body again, each time you pull towards you, you move down the spine (right).

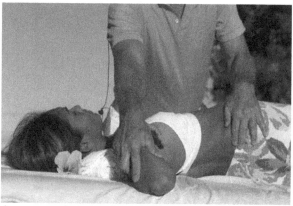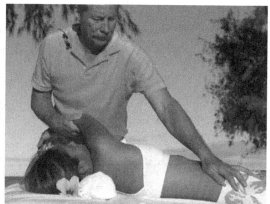

Just keep moving on down till you get to the hip (Left). The final time you place your hand on the anterior iliac crest and give one last stretch. I call this move giving the body a new pattern as you take them to an area they may have never stretched to...

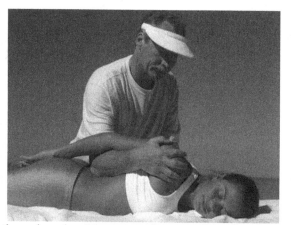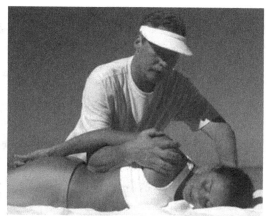

Another nice shoulder move is to reach under them and lift as my hand presses on the spine closest to me as I drop and move the hand as we go. Usually starting at the top of the back just below the neck.

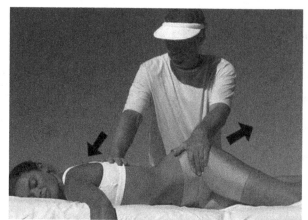

After the shoulder I move to this hips and now start to involve the whole spine, from, neck to shoulder to spine and end up in the hips. Lengthen the torso and all the muscles will follow.

CHAPTER TWENTY THREE
The Elbow

Medial Ligaments of the Elbow

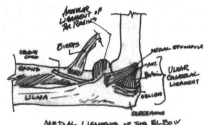

Lateral Ligaments of the Elbow

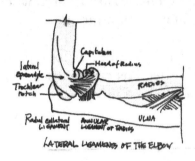

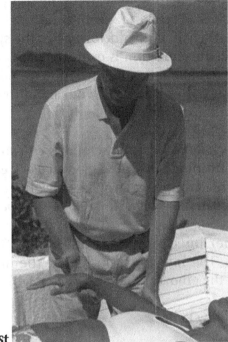

The test

The elbow is a rare place for an injury unless you play tennis, baseball or football. Three bones come together in this joint: the humerus, the ulna and the radius, as well as a capsule and a whole bunch of ligaments. The most common injury is what is called tennis elbow. It can be on the inside (medial) or the outside (lateral) of the joint. The muscles there on the lateral side are the extensors (see diagram of elbow for details). On the medial side, or inner side, of the elbow are the flexors. Carpenter's or tennis elbow pain runs from the elbow to the wrist, and at times it's painful on the medial (inside) side of the arm.

The problem with this injury is that it gets better as you play, and then it gets worse again. You can re-injure this tissue by playing again, since it seems that it feels better when you warm up, but then you feel it later and it's worse at night.

The test

Flex the hand at the elbow, and press on the dorsal part of the hand forcing it down. This stresses the extensor muscles and the pain will be felt right at the source of the injury, which is usually on the lateral side of the elbow on the radius muscle origin.

Treatment

RICE, or better MICE, is a good way to treat this injury. The ice bag on the elbow and the extension of the hand will accelerate the healing. Movement is important in this injury, because we want to reduce the adhesions, as these can cause further injury later. The key is to not use it in the way it was injured. Take a few weeks off your tennis game. If you re-injure the area, it can take months to get better.

DTF is one of the best ways to accelerate the healing. It will also break up the scar tissue formation. It will keep it from healing the wrong way causing future injury. The other approach is a corticosteroid injection. It has to be injected right into the exact point or it will not be effective. If the doctor misses the spot, the pain will return in a week or two. After the initial, acute condition is over, the best way to treat this injury is to strengthen the muscles. Use some dumbbells starting with five pounds. Support your arm and elbow on a table and with your palms down, lift your hand towards the ceiling extending the hand. After a few days work up to ten pound dumbbells.

If it's a chronic weak muscle, this can sometimes be from imbalanced muscles in the arm. Weight training is better when you use free weights. That way, all the peripheral muscles and supporting groups get stronger as well. These stabilizing muscles are injured when there is a weak one in the group. Remember, the weak link will always get injured.

The other injections are proliferants. They are good on chronic, or long-term, stubborn injuries. The injection will reduce the inflammation as well as create a scar tissue to help support the elbow at the joint, which will allow the body to heal the area.

Inner Elbow Pain

Pitcher's elbow or golfer's elbow are common names for this injury. Even some over use syndromes like vacuuming or house cleaning can create pain in this area. It's attached to the ulna and commonly called the funny bone. Once again, you may not even know what caused this injury to begin with, unless you are a pitcher, tennis player, or carpenter.

Test

To test this condition you flex your hand at the wrist, and the therapist pushes on the palm of the hand, forcing it dorsally (see picture).

Treatment

MICE is of course the treatment of choice during the acute phase. DTF is great for this area since the muscles are easy to get to. An old injury or a chronic condition will also respond to this treatment, although it will take much longer to help it get better.

A corticosteroid injection is helpful if the DTF does not make it better in a few weeks. It could take several injections to work. For the old and chronic injury, proliferant injections may be necessary to strengthen this tendon.

After the acute injury phase you need to strengthen the muscles by using dumbbells. Fix the arm resting your elbow on a table, the hand extended over the side, palm up, and flex the muscles while lifting the hand by bending the wrist. These exercises need to be kept up during the healing phase, too.

The best strategy would be to continue these exercises for life, particularly if you are doing something that stresses them to have caused the injury. In that case you need to keep them strong.

Arthritis of The Elbow

Arthritis is just another form of irritation, and lack of lubrication can cause this problem. It could come from over use or from nutritional deficiency as well. Usually injuries to the elbow can become chronic, or just worsen with time if not treated. This can lead to arthritis in any joint, for that matter. It then becomes more and more difficult to use the elbow, so that even opening up a jar of peanut butter hurts. You can get this from pitching 90 mile-an-hour baseballs, or by being a housewife washing the pots and pans. It's another of life's little mysteries why it can happen, and we need to look at the overall person once again.

The Test

Force the elbow to bend as far as it will go. When you try to straighten it, it will hurt just as badly. The ache can be constant, and of course, any movement will hurt.

Treatment

If it's a mild case, aspirin will help as will RICE along with the use of a sling. However, if it's not better in a couple of weeks, see a doctor. The worst thing to do, like with bursitis is to massage it, which will not help. RICE will only help for a few hours. It could take months to get better on its own after the acute phase.

The fastest treatment I have seen for this condition is injections of corticosteroid given a few days apart. Two or three treatments will do the trick. Wearing an arm sling will keep it less irritated, as movement will just increase the pain. No stretching or manipulations for this condition; you will make it worse and it will take twice as long to heal.

ROTATORS: The rotators, suppinate (rotate inward) and pronate (rotate outward)

Pronator Teres
Pronator Quadratus

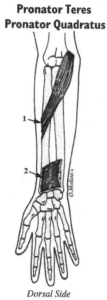

Dorsal Side

Pronator Teres

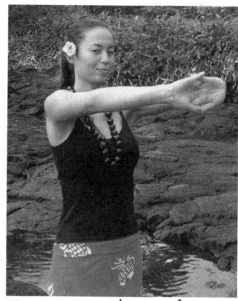

nice stretch

Origin: The lower part of the inner condyle ridge of the humerus and the medial side of the ulna.

Insertion: Middle third of the outer surface of the radius.

Action: Flexion of the forearm and pronation of the forearm as well.
Palpation is difficult because it is under the larger flexor group.

Strengthen: Use dumbbell curls, which work synergistically with the biceps group. Sometimes the origin is a very sore area, especially for athletes that use their hands with bats or rackets.

Massage: four sets of compression and DTF at the origin. This is a tender area so be careful.

Pronator Quadratus

Origin: The lower fourth of the anterior aspect of the ulna, just laterally.

Insertion: The lower fourth of the anterior aspect of the radius, just medially. It ties the two bones together at the wrist.

Action: Weak pronation of the forearm, in conjunction with the triceps brachii.

Supinator

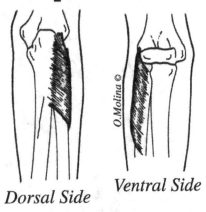

Dorsal Side   Ventral Side

Supinator (same stretch as above)

Origin: The outer condyloid ridge of the humerus and the neighboring part of the ulna, along the olecranon process of the ulna, next to triceps insertion.

Action: Straight suspiration of the forearm, for example, when opening a jar or turning a screwdriver.

Strengthening: Using dumbbells acts as a stabilizing force, to work it out you would need to do suppination with the weight resisting the action.

Massage: Mostly compression with the brachioradialis muscle and some deep friction is also effective, same as above.

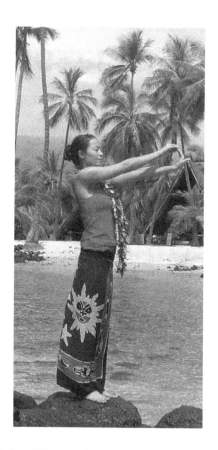

CHAPTER TWENTY FOUR
The Arm Flexors

The flexors and extensors of the fingers and the wrist encompass the whole forearm, the flexors located on the ventral (or underneath part) of forearm. Most of them originate at the medial epichondyle of the humerus. Picture Leilani shown lengthening the flexors, general stretch.

All the Flexors include:
Flexor carpi ulnaris (small finger); Flexor palmaris longus (palm); Flexor carpi radialis (closer to thumb); Flexor digitorum superficialis (superficial palm), and Flexor digitorum profundus (deep finger flexor).

Brachioradialis

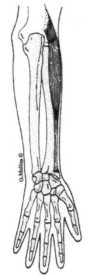

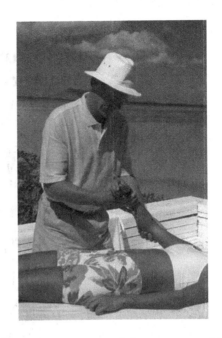

Brachioradialis Muscle   The test pull on wrist with arm at 90% lateral

Origin: Lower two thirds of the outer condyloid ridge of the humerus.

Insertion: The outer surface of the lower end of the radius at the styloid process.

Action: Flexion of the forearm, semi pronation and semi suppination.

Palpation: On the lateral anterior surface of the arm. It's the main muscle on the forearm, a third class lever. Because of its location it tends to pronate as it flexes. In a pronated position it tends to suppinate as it flexes. Common uses include baseball and tennis, and flexion of the arm works with the biceps as a stabilizer.

Stretching: Any form of extending the arm and rotating it.

Strengthening: Biceps curls with hand slightly supinated, as well as wrist curls.

Massage: Compression, cross fiber as well as deep longitudinal in the valleys.

Flexor Digitorum Superficialis

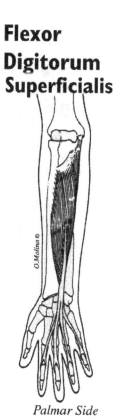

Palmar Side

Flexor Digitorum Sublimis

Origin: Inner condyle of the humerus, the ulna head medial coronoid area. As well, the radial head of the medial tuberosity.

Insertion: The tendons split and attach to the sides of the middle phalanx of the four fingers (palmar side).

Action: Flexes the fingers, wrist and forearm. All hand held sports.

Palpation: Anterior wrist surface on the ulna side, next to flexor carpi ulnaris.

Lengthen: Same as all the forearm muscles. See figures.

Strengthen: Wrist curls, stabilizer in weightlifting when using the hands and arms.

Flexor Pollicis Longus

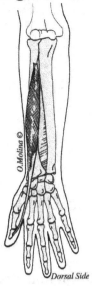

Dorsal Side

Flexor Pollicis Longus

Origin: Middle anterior surface of the medial head of the radius.

Insertion: The base of the distal phalanx of the thumb (palmar surface).

Action: true flexion of the thumb and the wrist.
A deep muscle, hard to palpate directly, work the same way as for all flexors.

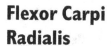

Flexor Carpi Radialis

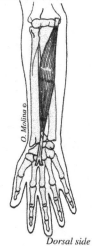

O. Molina ©

Dorsal side

Flexor Carpi Radialis/ Ulnaris

Origin: the inner condyle of the humerus.

Insertion: the base of the second and third metacarpals on the palmer surface.

Action: flexion of the wrist and the forearm.

Palpate the lower forearm on the ventral side, wiggle your fingers and you will feel the muscle.

Strengthen: by flexion with dumbbells, palm facing up. Important for tennis (forehand) or any hand held sports

Massage is always needed here, using compression four times in several areas. Then apply DTF at the origin and insertion; both areas are tender in most bodies. These have twice the use as the extensors do.

Flexor Carpi Ulnaris

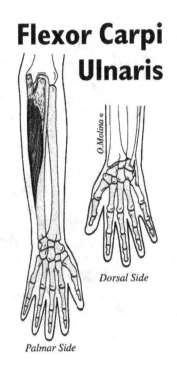

O.Molina

Dorsal Side

Palmar Side

Flexor Capri Ulnaris muscle

For the ulnaris, the only difference is that it inserts at the fifth metacarpal.

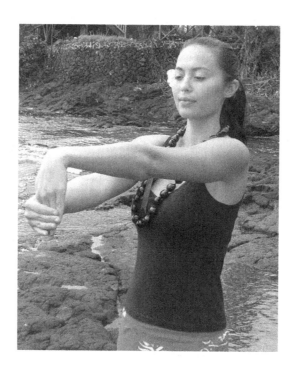

CHAPTER TWENTY FIVE
The Arm Extensors

The extensors are on the dorsal, or outside, part of the arm (Leilani shown lengthening them). They originate on the lateral epichondyle of the humerus, just opposite from the flexors. They are antagonistic to each other. They work in opposition or in unity, depending on the action. There are fewer extensors than flexors as you can see by the size of your arm. We're designed that way so that we can grip.

The extensors are, starting from the lateral, or outside, edge:
Extensor carpi ulnaris (off the ulna small finger); Extensor digiti minimi (ring finger); Extensor Digitorum (main fingers); Extensor indicis (underneath); Extensor Carpi radialis longus and brevis (off the radius, thumb and forefinger).

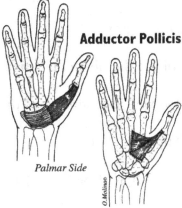

Abductor Pollicis Brevis

Adductor Pollicis

Palmar Side

O. Molinar

The Hand

The muscles acting on the thumb and the hand, they work in griping, both the flexors and extensors.

They are: Extensor pollicis longus (long one); Extensor pollicis brevis (short one); Abductor pollicis longus (pulls in long one), and Flexor pollicis longus (pulls to palm).

Movement of the thumb is very complex and involves many muscles working together. Many insert in very close positions, but because of the layout they do slightly different actions. The ulnar eminence, palmer side of thumb. The muscles are Opponecus pollicis; Abductor pollicis brevis, and Flexor pollicis brevis.

The Hypothenar Eminence (palmar side, small finger). Those muscles are: Opponens digiti minimi, Flexor digiti minimi brevis, and Abductor digiti minimi. These muscles work with the thumb in gripping and grasping actions.

The deep muscles of the hand (palmar side) are: Adductor pollicis, Palmar interosseous, Dorsal interosseous and Lumbricals. All these muscles work in concert to grasp, to write, and to do the many other complex actions the hand and fingers do.

Stretching: For these hand muscles you interlace your fingers and turn palms out with arms extended out in front of you. Strengthening these muscles takes squeezing a rubber ball, or any weightlifting holding, because these are stabilizer muscles.

Massage: For the flexors and extensors massage is very much the same. Compression on the belly of the muscle is very beneficial. So is cross fiber with or without oil. For injuries or for the tendons, DTF is recommended.

Stretch: Interlace fingers for the flexors and stretch with arms out in front. For the extensors, stretch by bending the wrist with the other hand to increase the length in the extensor group.

Strengthen: Arm curls and extension, working with dumbbells. Also, any heavy lifting using free weights, where the arms are directly involved.

Extensor Pollicis Longus

Origin: At the upper posterior surface of the ulna.

Insertion: the base of the last phalanx of the thumb on the dorsal surface.

Action: Primary extension of the wrist as well as extension of the thumb.

Palpate: Touch as you move the thumb up and down.

Strengthen: With some wrist curls moving the wrist with the palms horizontal. Raising thumb towards the direction of the radius.

Massage: As with all the flexors compression and DTF are great for this type of muscle.

**Extensor Carpi
Radialis Brevis**

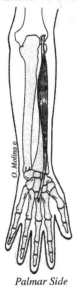

Palmar Side

Extensor Carpi Radialis Brevis

Origin: External condyle of the humerus.

Insertion: Base of the third metacarpal (the dorsal surface).

Action: Extension of the wrist and extension of the forearm.

Palpation: Dorsal side of the forearm. Find the elbow at the medial external condyle of the humerus and flex your wrist. You will feel the origin.

Lengthen: Flex the arm with elbow straight.

Strengthen: Good for tennis elbow, from improper backhand. Hold dumbbell, fix elbow with palm down, flex wrist and lift weight towards ceiling.
Uses: Backhand in tennis, swinging a baseball bat, part of a golf swing. Any action that uses the wrist in a cocking action.

Massage: Compression, as well as some cross fiber work to loosen and lengthen. A very good area for trigger point and acupressure location.

Extensor Carpi Ulnaris

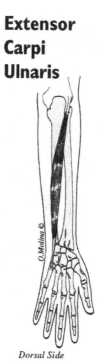

Dorsal Side

Extensor Carpi Ulnaris

Origin: Lateral condyle of the humerus. Posterior proximal ridge of the ulna.

Insertion: Base of the fifth metacarpal bone (on the dorsal side)

Action: Extension of the wrist, and adduction with the flexor carpi ulnaris muscle. Extension of the forearm (backhand in tennis).

Palpation: Insertion at the anterior ulna side of the forearm, on the fifth metacarpal.

Lengthen: The same as extensor carpi radialis. They work together as well. Flexors of the arm and wrist.

CHAPTER TWENTY SIX
Muscles Of The Shoulder

Deltoid Group

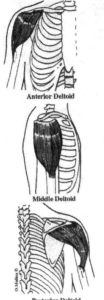

Deltoids

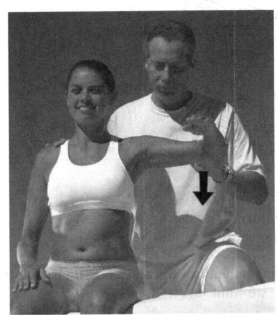

Deltoids Test: Stabilize other shoulder, push down on elbow.

Origin: Anterior outer third of the clavicle, the acromion process, and the superior lateral edge of the spine of the scapula.

Insertion: The deltoideus tubercle, on the middle of the outer surface of the humerus, a half way distal from the shoulder joint.

Action: True abduction, the whole fibers, with some anterior (flexion, with inward rotation) and some posterior action (extension, with outward rotation) when used separate. The deltoids also works with the trapezius to fix the scapula allowing the humerus to be the lever to abduct the arm. All lifting movements using the arms, especially sideways.

Palpation: It caps the shoulder, over the head of the humerus and the lateral edge of the clavicle and scapular spine.

Strengthen: Lifting dumbbells, straight up with the arms extended out. Machine variations include some with the arms bent, using the elbows to lift the pads. Military presses also work these muscles as well as pulley systems, when abduction of the arms is used.

Massage: These muscles are often stressed as well, the whole shoulder area is often tight and overworked. Especially if not mechanically aligned. Compression is always a good way to warm up a muscle, without oil. Circular massage is a gentle way to start, and then gentle oil strokes with the fibers, as well as across the fibers. DTF can be done and is very effective at the origin and insertion, as this is usually the site for injuries.

Pectoralis Major

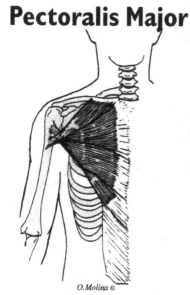

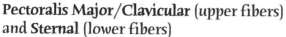

Pectoralis Major/Clavicular (upper fibers) and Sternal (lower fibers)

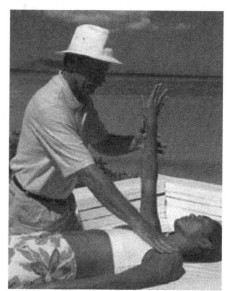

The Test for Pectoralis

Origin: The medial half of the clavicle. The lateral border of the sternum as well as the top six ribs at the sternum.

Insertion: It becomes a flat tendon at the distal end of the muscle and attaches to the humerus at the inter tubercular groove.

Action: Flexion (clavicular) Draws the arm forward and upward from the side. Extends the arm further upward especially after it's above the shoulder level. Horizontal Flexion (middle fibers) draws the arm forward from a side horizontal position to the front of the body (forward). Inward rotation and adduction can draw the arm down and across the chest and lower (sternal inferior fibers). It also slightly rotates the humerus inward.

Palpate across the chest.

Strengthen: Push ups, bench press, flies, any kind of pressing weights using the hands in front of the chest. The lower fibers work in conjunction with the latissimus dorsi when adducting the humerus. Other antagonists are the infraspinatus and the teres major.

Lengthen: Pulling the arms back as far as possible, interlacing the fingers behind the back. Hanging can stretch it as can holding on to a door frame and stretching the body forward, hands behind you.

Massage across the chest or in circles (For women, work above the breast not on them. The breasts are only fatty tissue, so they don't need massage.) Cross fiber on these muscles is excellent, as they too seem to be tense areas.

For injuries, see different muscle tests for these muscles, and apply DTF. Some compression can also be used in this area.

Pectoralis Minor

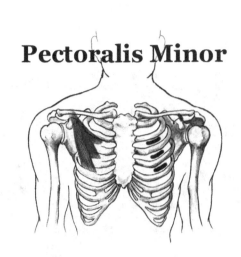

Pectoralis Minor

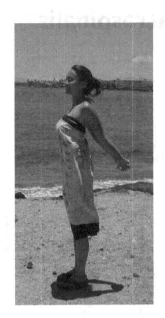

Good pectoralis stretch

Origin: Outer surface of the third, fourth, and fifth rib just lateral from the sternum, close to where the origin of the serratus anterior is, making it a stabilizer muscle in the action of push ups or any heavy shoulder and scapula action.

Insertion: The coracoid process of the scapula.

Action: True abduction of the scapula, draws the scapula forward and tilts the inferior border of the scapula away from the ribs. Works in opposition to the rhomboids muscle, as it acts in adduction of the scapula. The rhomboid is its antagonist along with lower trapezius muscles. It's stabilized by the serratus anterior, together they pull together in true abduction, which is necessary in push ups. They stabilize each other, one pulling back as well as down and the other one forward and upward.

Palpation: Only felt close to the insertion at the coracoid process, when arm is raised and you exert pressure downward. Adduction of the arm will cause the muscle to be palpated just medial of the greater tubercle of the humerus in the pit just inferior to the distal end of the clavicle.

Strengthen: Most push ups, bench press, any action involving the pectoralis group and the shoulder action.

Massage: This area is difficult to reach, as it's under the pectoralis major, which is much larger. You can work on it near the insertion. Cross fiber massage is great for this muscle as it is often tight and stressed. The shoulder is often a site for tension, and massage of this area is critically important. (See pectoralis massage and therapy.)

Sacrospinalis

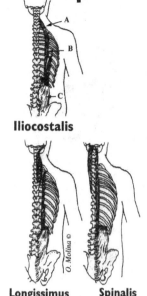

Iliocostalis

O. Molina ©

Longissimus   **Spinalis**

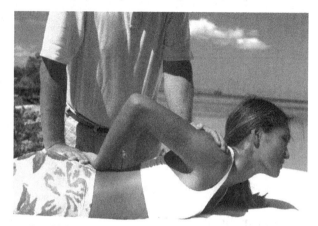

Erector Spinae muscle (Sacrospinalis)   **Test: Push on shoulder on each side.**

Origin: The posterior crest of the ilium, the lower posterior surface of the sacrum. The inferior border of the angles of the lower seven ribs. The spinous process of all the lumbar and the lower four thoracic vertebrae. Transverse processes of all the thoracic vertebrae.

Insertion: The angles of the ribs, the transverse process of all the vertebrae and the base of the skull toward the mastoid process. Obviously, this muscle weaves itself though the whole spine and rib cage, completing the basket around the rib cage.

Action: Extension of the spine and some extension of the neck (help to bring the head backwards). Works with the abdominal muscles in holding the trunk together, and with core movements.

Strengthen: Dead man lift, holding dumbbells or barbells in hand, bending over and using the back muscles and gluts to stand up.

Massage: Because these are such complex muscles, it's critical to do very detailed work with them. Work like compression is very effective. Deep Swedish or massage along the muscles of the back is done in every culture. Then working with DTF, knowing where the muscles are, and being very specific, you get many areas of tension in this muscle group.

Supraspinatus

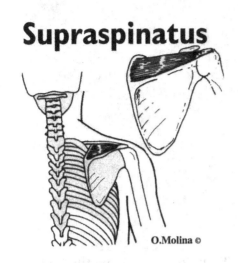

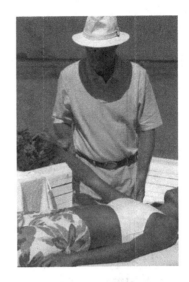

Supraspinatus Muscle

The test push towards groin arm at 40%

O.Molina ©

Origin: The supraspinatus fossa, a grove just superior to the spinous process of the scapula.

Insertion: The top of the greater tubercle of the humerus.

Action: Weak abduction, fires initially in the first 30% before the deltoids take over. It works with the deltoids as in throwing. A first class lever helps hold the humerus in the glenoid fossa socket).

Strengthen: BY working with the deltoids it's strengthened by abduction of the arms as with dumbbells, military press, latissimus pulls, and some shrugs as well.

Lengthen: Moving the arm behind the small of your back and increasing the pull of the arm on the shoulder. Also, holding the elbows and stretching arm across the chest as for the triceps.

Massage: It's hard to get in there because the trapezius muscle is over the top. You can always do your four sets of compression. If it's injured you can do DTF, locating the painful site with a test and following with the friction massage. You can at times work the insertion, as it's on the posterior aspect of the greater tubercle of the humerus.

Latissimus Dorsi

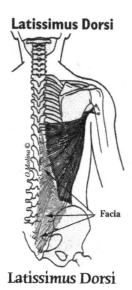

Latissimus Dorsi

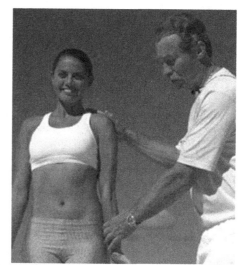

Test: Pull away from the body.

Origin: Posterior crest of the iliac spine, the upper portion of the sacrum, the lower five thoracic vertebrae, the spinous process of the lumbar vertebra and just a touch at the lower three ribs.

Insertion: Medial and inner side of the greater inter tubercular groove of the humerus (just superior of the pectoralis muscles group).

Action: Extension, drawing the arm from a front horizontal position down to the side as with the pectoralis. Along with inward rotation as it draws the arm in and down, it helps to stabilize the arm action with the pectoralis group.
Horizontal extension like the pectoralis also draws the arm from the front to the side position. Its main job is adduction, drawing the arm from the side horizontal position down to the side, it rotates inward as it adducts. The true antagonist is the pectoralis major sternal, along with some of the posterior deltoids and the teres minor and infraspinatus.

Strengthen: Any type of rowing involves this muscle, pull downs on pulleys, overhead pull ups, as well as some work when you are doing push ups and bench presses. Also, it's a very important swimming muscle.

Palpation: Not hard to find: the whole lower half of the back.

Massage to this muscle is also very important. Long, deep strokes with the spine will give you cross fiber on the muscle. Also, massage with the grain for drainage. Most important, at the back of the muscle along the spine is a large sheet of fascia. This is a tight area on most people; use the elbows to get a deep stroke. It is rarely injured, except by competitive paddling or it becomes strained by swimming.

202

Teres Major

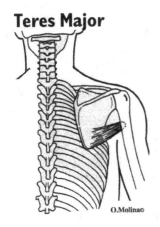

O.Molina©

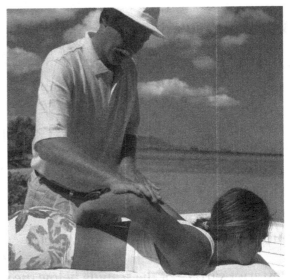

Teres Major Test

Origin: Lower third of the lateral border of the scapula.

Insertion: The inner edge of the inter tubercular grove of the humerus, just inferior to the latissimus insertion, and medially from the pectoralis group.

Action: Extension, works with the latissimus, in moving the arm from the front down to the side of the body, with inward rotation as it moves down. Adduction from the side horizontal position down to the side of the body. It's only effective for this action when the rhomboids is fixed, and is the assistant to the

Strengthen: Any type of rowing involves this muscle, pull downs on pulleys, overhead pull ups, as well as some work when you are doing push ups and bench presses. Also, it's a very important swimming muscle.

Palpation: Not hard to find: the whole lower half of the scapula.

Massage: cross fiber and trigger points are great for this muscle it is usually sore be careful.

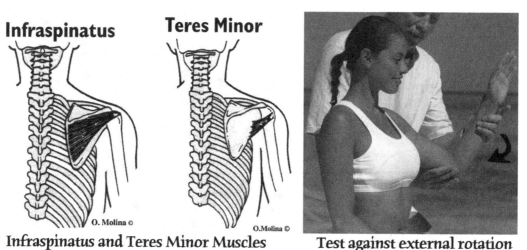

Infraspinatus   **Teres Minor**

O. Molina ©   O.Molina ©

Infraspinatus and Teres Minor Muscles   **Test against external rotation**

Origin: Posterior surface of the scapula below the spine and medial border.

Insertion: Greater tubercle of the humerus on the posterior side.

Action: Horizontal extension, it draws the humerus from the front position to the side position. Another extension, it also draws the humerus from the front horizontal position down to the side of the body. It rotates outward as it extends or depresses the scapula. Its antagonist is the pectoralis major as it attaches on the anterior part of the greater tubercle of the humerus. The rhomboids also stabilize it.

Strengthen and Lengthen: All the same rowing and posterior shoulder work.

Massage: For this area, the same as all the circle work around the shoulder and scapula, up medially and inferior laterally. DTF can be done very effectively on these muscles, in fact, you will find many trigger points as well.

Subscapularis

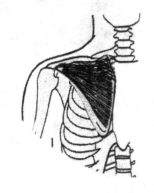

Subscapularis Muscle

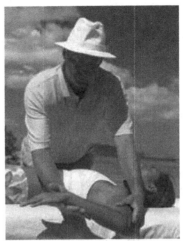

The test

Origin: The anterior medial subscapularis fossa, on the rib side of the scapula, and medial border.

Insertion: The lesser tubercle of the humerus medially to the pectoralis insertion, this is also a stabilizer.

Action: Extension draws the humerus from the front horizontal position down to the side. Rotation inward as it depresses.
Adduction: draws the arm down to the side from the side horizontal position and rotates inward as it adducts. Antagonists are the pectoralis muscles as well as teres minor and infraspinatus, and even some teres major action. It helps hold the head of the humerus in the glenoid fossa, and it works with the latissimus dorsi and teres major because of the proximity to the joint.

Strengthen with all the latissimus and with rowing workout.

Massage is impossible as it's on the costal side of the scapula.

Trapezius

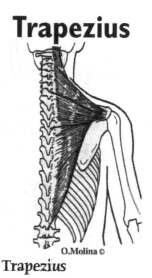

Trapezius

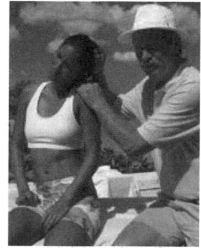

More of an upper trapezius test

Origin: Base of the skull at the occipital protuberance, and some of the ligaments on the posterior part of the neck. The spinous process of the seventh and all the thoracic vertebrae. It also interweaves with the supraspinatus ligaments on the spine.

Insertion: Posterior aspect of the lateral third of the clavicle. The lateral border of the acromion process and the upper border of the spine of the scapula.

Action: It elevates the scapula and acts with the rhomboid muscle to adduct the scapula. Its typical action is upward rotation of the scapula. In moving the arms to an overhead position the muscle rotates the scapula upward. Antagonist is the pectoralis minor.

Palpation: It's one of the larger muscles on the back and it works in most arm held exercises and shoulder movements. It's a third class lever, and along with the pectoral muscles and the sternoclavicular joint, it creates a pivot point for the shoulder.

Strengthening: Shrugs with dumbbells, in conjunction with latissimus on rowing, and in military presses with the deltoids and pectoralis major clavicular.

Lengthening: Along with the triceps, any type of arm pulling across the chest, as well as holding on to something fixed with the hands and stretching the body back to lengthen the thoracic spine.

Massage: Massaging the back in any form is bound to work on the trapezius. Some of the best work comes in following the origin to insertion (Swedish, lymphatic cleansing) as well as some very specific cross fiber massage on the whole length of the fibers. Circles around the scapula are very effective.

Rhomboids :
Minor & major

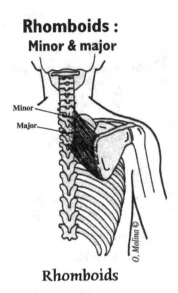

Minor

Major

O. Molina ©

Rhomboids

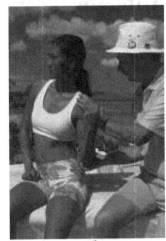

The test

Origin: The spinous processes of the last cervical and the first five thoracic vertebrae.

Insertion: The medial border of the scapula, below the spinous ridge.

Action: Adduction of the scapula (draws the scapula towards the spine) and with the trapezius elevates slightly as it adducts. It also rotates the scapula downwards, when the arms are up, in the action with the latissimus dorsi. The antagonist is the serratus anterior. Its action is to adduct the scapula, when you extend the arms. It also works in drawing the border of the scapula medially when the latissimus dorsi comes into play. Along with the triceps, it works in the crawl stroke in swimming.

Palpation: It's hard to feel directly as it's under the trapezius muscle. It's also a third class lever.

Strengthen: Bent over reverse flies, as well as any rowing movements, and in any arm movement that works in opposition to any pectoralis work, in conjunction with the trapezius muscle, and some latissimus dorsi action. Its antagonist is the serratus anterior and teres major as a stabilizer. Also works in chin ups, or pull downs on a pulley system.

Lengthen: Same action as trapezius, any arm lengthening, and hanging from a bar.

207

Anterior Serratus

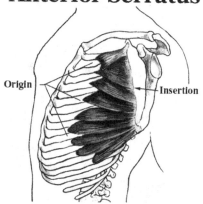

Anterior Serratus Muscle

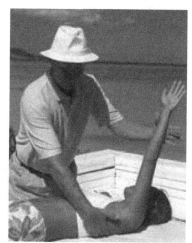

Test for Anterior Serratus

These muscles along with the serratus posterior are very complex muscles that weave between the ribs.

Origin: The surface of the upper nine ribs and the lateral side of the sternum.

Insertion: The costal aspect of the medial border of the scapula, just opposite from where the rhomboids insertion is. Thus it's antagonistic since they have opposite actions.

Action: Draws the medial border of the scapula away from the vertebrae, abduction. Provides some upward rotation of the inferior border of the scapula. Works with the pectoralis muscles in arm movements like throwing a ball.

Palpation: Lateral anterior side of the chest, just below the fifth and sixth ribs.

Strengthen: To strengthen you can do push ups, in pulleys you could use the arm motion pulling the arm across the chest, or pull downs involving the latissimus dorsi. If you suspect weakness in this muscle it's easy to test. Have patient push against a wall, and if their scapula turns on edge, they have a weak anterior serratus.

Lengthen: Hanging, or any movement opening up the arms away from the chest.

Massage is done with strokes moving from just lateral of the sternum, following the ribs laterally and superior to the arm pit. Sometimes these muscles can get micro-tears or injuries where you have to test them and find the lesion. Then DTF massage is very effective if you find the precise area

CHAPTER TWENTY SEVEN
The Abdominals

Rectus Abdominis

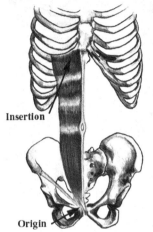

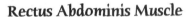

Rectus Abdominis Muscle

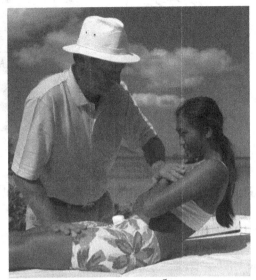

The test

Origin: The superior crest of the pubis. The origin and insertion can be switched depending on the movement. We are speaking from a sitting up position as movement.

Insertion: Cartilage of the fifth, sixth, and seventh ribs and the xiphoid process, at the base of the sternum. There are two sections, divided by the linea alba, in the center of the abdominals.

Action: Flexion and lateral flexion of the trunk. It also pulls down on the ribs to stabilize the whole anterior section of the body.

Strengthen: The best way is by doing crunchies, straight ahead and to each side, and for the oblique group (laterally), diagonal crunchies. The abs are critical for allowing the hip flexors to work more effectively. It's abdominal weakness that leads to causing all the other muscles over work and stress the low back. When they are weak, they make the psoas tight and act up. We often confuse the symptom (low back problems) with the actual problem (tight psoas).

Massage: All the massage for the abdominals is much the same; it's not a vitally complex technique. (See specific massage.)

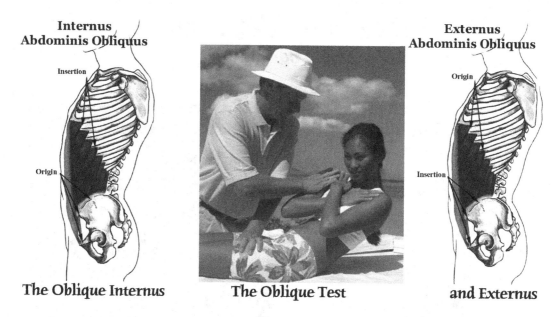

Internus Abdominis Obliquus — Insertion — Origin

Externus Abdominis Obliquus — Origin — Insertion

The Oblique Internus   **The Oblique Test**   **and Externus**

The way these two muscles differ is that their origins and insertions are reversed.

Externus

Origin: Borders of the lower eight ribs at the side of the chest dovetailing in with the serratus anterior. They also, in a way, create a basket of muscle around the whole chest cavity, with the serratus posterior bringing up the rear.

Insertion: The front half of the crest of the ilium, the inguinal ligament, the crest of the pubis and the fascia of the rectus abdominis muscle at the inferior end of the linea alba.

Action: Flexes the trunk. The right side of the muscle contraction makes you twist left, and the left side contraction makes your body twist to the right. They do this twisting action working independently. Of course, when they work together then they act as the rectus muscle.

Internus

Origin: The upper half of the inguinal ligament (superior), anterior two-thirds of the rest of the ilium and the lumbar fascia. Attaches at the inferior lateral border of the diamond lumbar fascia (a site for deep therapy).

Insertion: The costal cartilages of the eighth, ninth, and tenth ribs and the linea alba.

Action: Right side flexes your torso to the right, and the left to the left.

Transversus Abdominis Muscle

Origin: The outer third of the inguinal ligament, the inner rim of the crest of the ilium, as well as the surface of the lower six ribs. It also ties into the lumbar fascia.

Insertion: The crest of the pubis and the iliopectineal line and the linea alba.

Action: This is the muscle that holds in the abdomen, and when you exhale with force you contract this muscle. Isometrics is a good way to strengthen all the abdominals.

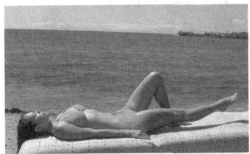 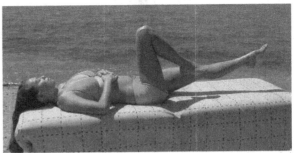

Gentle simple ways to start to strengthen your abdominals (Left) one leg at a time (right) both legs working. Always make sure and contract your abs.

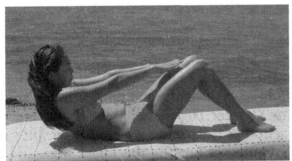 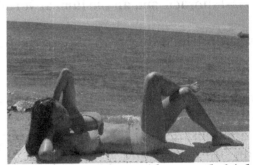

Next level up is crunchies for rectus abdominals (left) transverse side to side crunch (right). Do both sides never pull head pull at the neck. Easy!

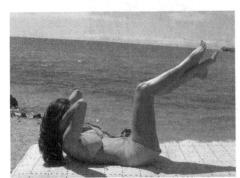 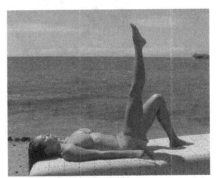

Crunchies variation legs high.   Circles with both legs great stabilizer.

Psoas & Iliacus

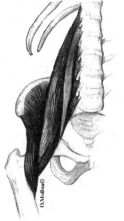

Iliopsoas Muscle

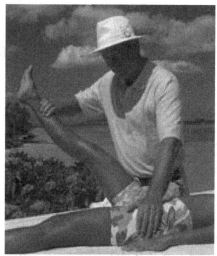

The Test

Origin: Inner (ventral) surface of the ilium, the base of the sacrum, and sides of the bodies of the last thoracic and all the lumbar vertebrae.

Insertion: The lesser trochanter of the femur and the shaft of the femur below.

Action: Flexion of the thigh at the hip and outward rotation of the thigh. When the thigh is fixed, the psoas muscle pulls on the vertebrae and flexes the spine and the pelvis to a sitting position. It raises the legs when you are lying supine. This is why when working the abdominals; it's best to get the psoas out of the action by flexing the legs. (crunchies) It's the main hip flexor, and gets strengthened by running with kicking the knees high and by certain sit ups. Pilates work can improve the abdominal functioning with this muscle. Antagonist is the gluteus group; sometimes the iliacus is its partner.

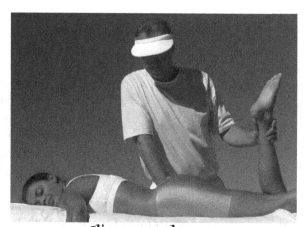

Iliacus muscle test:
Hold at a 90 degree angle below the ankle and rotate outwards (External rotation)

212

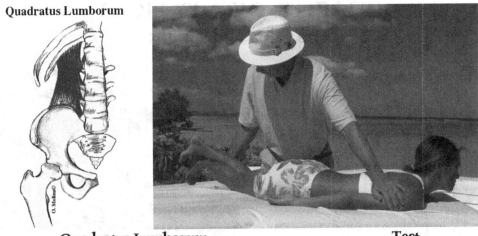

Quadratus Lumborum

Quadratus Lumborum   Test

Origin: Posterior inner lip of the iliac crest and transverse processes of the lower four lumbar vertebrae.

Insertion: the transverse processes of the upper two lumbar vertebrae and the lower border of the twelfth rib.

Action: Extension of the lower back when both are used together. It does lateral flexion when used one at a time. Works synergistically with the abdominals and erector spinae muscle (Sacrospinalis).

Massage: It's hard to get at, yet it is a very commonly stressed muscle. This gives some soothing relief to it, along with any work on the gluteus group as well as the erectors of the whole back area.

Test: With the patient prone and bent towards you, the object is to spread the body apart. It's tricky and it takes some time to get used to this test, but don't worry, it's not used very often.

CHAPTER TWENTY EIGHT
The Hips and Thighs

Hip Flexors & Facia lata

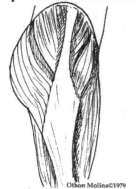

Othon Molina©1979

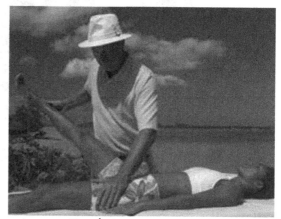

Fascia Lata test

Injuries

Most injuries to the hips are due to misalignment of the pelvis. The torque can aggravate several areas, most commonly the hip at the trochanter where the femur meets this hip joint and is a stressful area. You can get trochanter bursitis as there is a bursa at the head of the femur, and it can be a painful situation. For this condition only an injection can help, as massage will irritate it further.

The muscles involved there are the insertion of the gluteus group and the fascia lata. One of the muscles involved is often the periformis. This deep gluteal muscle can have a lot of stress put on it if the pelvis is out of alignment. In fact, most runners have tension and some tightness in the gluteal muscles since these are the main hip extensors and are used in running, jumping, and most sports.

They seldom are injured as far as a tear occurring because they are very strong muscles. But they can become stressed because of over use syndrome. Most runners get stressed there from long distance training. You can also get injured here in contact sports or from falling on the hip. Other injuries can happen to the ligaments holding the hip to the sacrum, and these can be a problem (see back). Weightlifters doing heavy squats can hurt this area. Also, moving in the wrong direction or a fall on the buttocks, are ways to injure these ligaments.

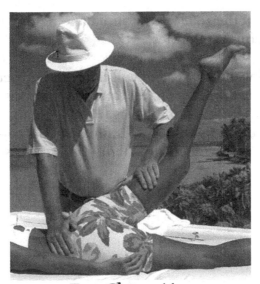

Test: Gluteus Max

For injuries to the gluteus group, test the gluteus maximus. With the patient prone, have them lift the knee off the table. Stabilize the opposite hip and press down on the back of the hamstring. If this hurts it will be noticeable in the tissue that's injured. If it's more at the front of the hip, have them sitting and lift the knee towards the ceiling while you push down on the thigh and resist the movement (hip flexors test).

If the muscle pain is more on the side, then have them lie with the painful side up while on their side and abduct the leg (raise the leg off the table). Have them hold and you push down at the knee. If that hurts it could be the fascia lata muscle. If you still can find the injury location, do the periformis test: Patient supine, bend the knee 90% and have them move the leg medially while you push laterally at the ankle. (External rotation of the hip)

For the ligaments, have the patient supine. Then move the leg on the suspected side over to the opposite pelvis, and put a stretch on the ligaments. Palpation is next. Press on the lateral edge of the sacrum, and feel for pain. It can be very painful to the touch.

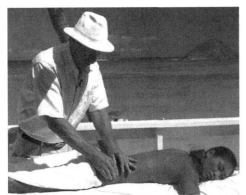
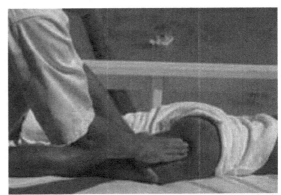

TREATMENT: Gluteus Massage Stroke (left) compression (right)

RICE of course is the treatment of choice, unless it's in the deeper gluteus muscles. The next approach is DTF massage on the lesion. You can also use compression massage for the gluteus group. Further down the road, work on balancing the pelvis as well as deep cross friction massage to prevent further injuries.

The ligaments will respond well to DTF, and will improve in three to four weeks. Be careful not to stretch this area during the acute phase. Later they may respond well to manipulations of the sacroiliac joint (SI joint). For the ligaments, if all else fails an injection of corticosteroid can increase the healing. For stubborn and consistent pain in the sacral ligaments, a proliferant injection will create stability and scar tissue to aid in the healing.

Gluteus Maximus

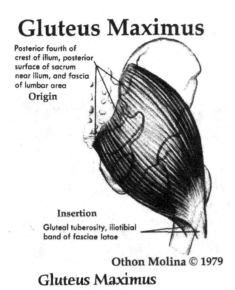

Posterior fourth of crest of ilium, posterior surface of sacrum near ilium, and fascia of lumbar area
Origin

Insertion
Gluteal tuberosity, iliotibial band of fasciae latae

Othon Molina © 1979

Gluteus Maximus

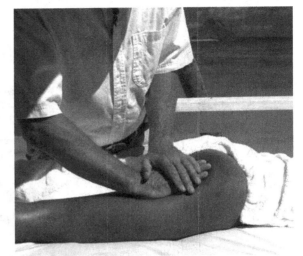

Compression on Gluteus

The gluteus is one of the most important of all muscles. Running, jumping, and just getting up all engage extension of the leg at the hip.

Origin: Posterior fourth of the crest of the iliac spine. The posterior surfaces of the sacrum near the ilium and the fascia of the whole lumbar area.

Insertion: The gluteal tuberosity of the femur and the iliotibial band of the fascia latae.

Action: Extension of the thigh at the hip. Outward rotation of the thigh, as well as some adduction with the lower fibers. One of the most important running muscles as well as major leg extension.

Lengthen: Down on the floor with legs bent, lean chest towards knees (focuses on the deep gluteus muscles). Lying on back, knee to chest stretches the gluts as well as the low back. Use caution with this stretch, it's not recommended when disc injury is present.

Strengthening: Squats with weights on shoulder or in hands, lunging, jumping or any running up hills. It works in conjugation with the hamstring group.

Massage: Compression is great on these muscles. Relaxing the gluteals is very important. Massage with this muscle relaxes the low back. Deep circles with the upward stroke on the medial side and down on the lateral side. Cross fiber follows the sacrum.

Gluteus Medius

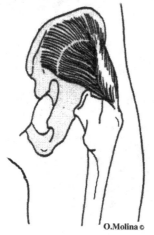

Gluteus Medius

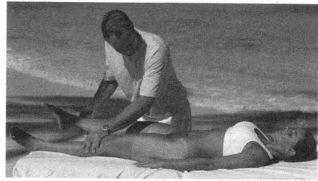

The Test

Origin: Superior and the outer surface of the ilium just below posterior to the iliac crest.

Insertion: The posterior medial surface of the greater trochanter of the femur.

Action: This is any kind of abduction of the thigh, with some outward rotation. Anther running muscle works, with the gluts with same stretching and strengthening.

Strengthen: Squats, lunges, anything that works the legs through to the gluts.

Lengthen: Sit on floor, with leg bent under you and bend towards your knee.

Gluteus Minimus

Origin: Outer surface of the ilium below the origin of the medius.

Insertion: Anterior surface of the greater trochanter of the femur.

Action: Abduction of the femur on the pelvis, with some inward rotation as well. Works with the maximus, medius, and deep gluteals.

Strength, Lengthen, and Massage: The same as with all the gluteals.

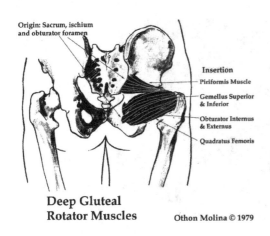

Origin: Sacrum, ischium and obturator foramen

Insertion
Piriformis Muscle
Gemellus Superior & Inferior
Obturator Internus & Externus
Quadratus Femoris

Deep Gluteal Rotator Muscles

Othon Molina © 1979

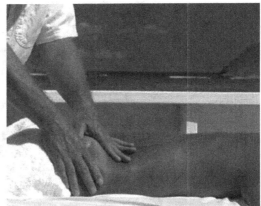

Massage for Gluteus Medius

The Deep Gluteals: Periformis, Gemellus, Obturator and Quadratus Femoris

Origin: Sacrum, posterior aspect of the ischium and obturator foramen.
Insertion: Greater trochanter and the posterior aspect of the greater trochanter.

Action: Lateral rotation, these muscles stabilize the running wheels and the front thigh and hamstring group. Also used in deep hip motion, as in batting, leading with the hips or martial arts.

Strengthen: Working the gluteals in the same way, as well as lengthening and massage.

To me, the basis of the whole body alignment is the pelvis. If the pelvis is rotated, the spine as well as the back and neck are under stress (physical and structural). Massage gives just temporary relief if you do not align the pelvis. The key is to determine the existing alignment, if one hip is superior to the other, as well as the anterior rotation. The place to measure is the superior anterior iliac spine, right in the notch. Hold fingers pointing medial and determine which side is anterior. Start with the anterior hip always. If it's anterior superior the move is as follows:

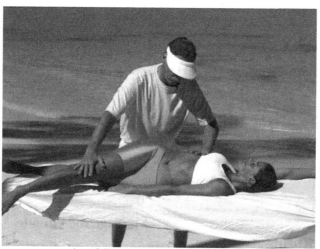

Superior hip being stretched inferior.

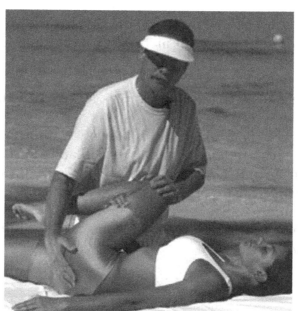

Inferior hip stretched superior, and towards the opposite shoulder

All the work is being done on the sacro-iliac ligaments so it should be done slow and easy. Some cross fiber massage on the ligaments and muscles is helpful to get the full range of the exercise. Patients may do this on their own to accelerate the alignment of the hips.

Semimembranosus

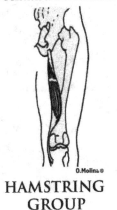

HAMSTRING GROUP

Semitendinosus

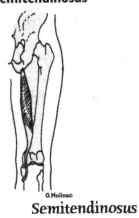

Semitendinosus

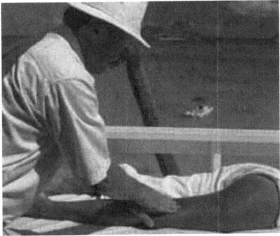

Muscle Massage

Origin: The inferior tuberosity of the ischium (right next to its other hamstring buddy).

Insertion: The upper anterior medial condyle of the tibia.

Action: Extension of the thigh at the hip, one of the three in the hamstring group. Flexion of the leg at the knee as well as outward rotation of the femur (External Rotation). Works with the gluteus maximus in running, jumping, etc.

Strengthen: By squats, lunges, and deep knee bends as they work in extension of the hip. However, weights are much more effective for this particular group.

Lengthening: This muscle group is critical for effective running as well as for less stress on the low back.

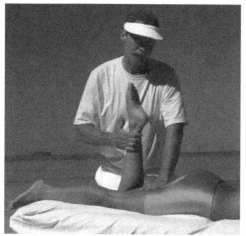 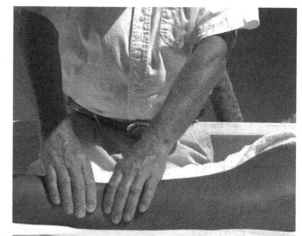

The General Hamstring Muscle Test   Semimembranosus muscle friction

Origin: The most lateral tuberosity of the ischium, right next to other hamstring member.

Insertion: The posterior surface of the medial condyle of the tibia.

Action: Extension of the thigh at the hip, one of the three in the hamstring group. Flexion of the leg at the knee, as well as inward rotation of the femur (Internal Rotation). Works with the gluteus maximus in running, jumping, etc.

Strengthen: By squats, lunges, deep knee bends, as they do work in extension of the hip. However, weights are much more effective for this particular group.

Lengthening; This muscle group is critical for effective running as well as for less stress on the low back.

Massage: See hamstring group. Deep at the origin on left and across the insertion on right.
HAMSTRINGS

These muscles at the back of the leg are very often injured in track and field, or in football. In fact, any all out running sport can injure a hamstring. The actual muscles we are talking about are the biceps femoris, the vastus laterals, semimembranosus, and the semitendinosus. I have heard this injury make a very loud pop. Often it's because of improper warm-up. It can also be caused because the quads are so much stronger that the balance becomes out of proper control. Often the quads are twice as strong as the hamstrings, and it should be closer ratio of 60:40. It can hurt in the buttocks, all over the back of the thigh, or at the knee.

Test for Hamstrings

Have the patient lie prone; have them bend the knee, till the foot is straight up in the air. Support the hamstrings as you pull down at the ankle. This will set off the pain and give you a clue as to where the injury is. These muscles heal quickly, but you have to make sure you get them treated right, NO STRETCHING.

Treatment

MICE is great for healing this injury, the sooner the better. You may have seen football games where there is a guy with an ice bag and an ace bandage standing on the sidelines. You can reduce the healing time by days if you ice it right away. Keep it moving too, which will create a subtle scar tissue and keep it flexible.

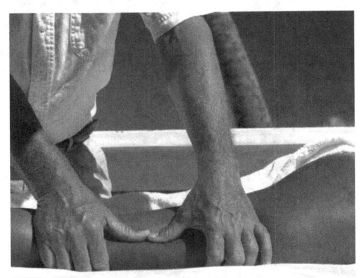

DTF on Insertion of the Hamstrings Lateral Aspect.

DTF is the best on these tissues as they are easy to get to and will respond well to the therapy. Later you can do deep tissue massage to increase circulation and separate the muscles from each other. The key is to not let an improper scar tissue form there or you can have a chronic injury. Many runners hurt it over and over again because they don't get the proper treatment. You will see a big hematoma on it in a day or two. You can still work on it, just be careful. If left alone, it will heal in three to four weeks if it's not severe. However, it can plague an athlete for years if it heals improperly. Injury prevention is by strengthening them with weight training; do twice the workout on the hamstrings that you do on the quadriceps. Lunges are also a good way to strengthen, as well as lengthen, the hamstring group.

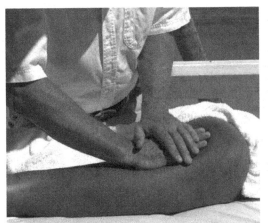 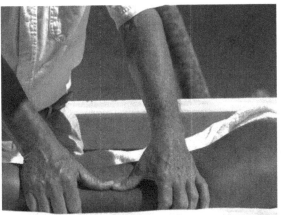

Above some compression on the origin of the hamstrings (left). Then cross fiber work on the tendons of the semimembranosis, lateral side of hamstrings (Right)

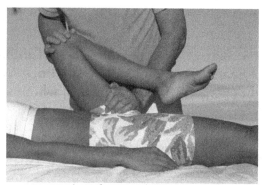 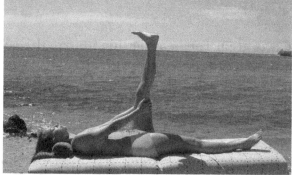

⁃   An assisted stretch for the hamstrings gentle.   Self stretch more intense, go slow.

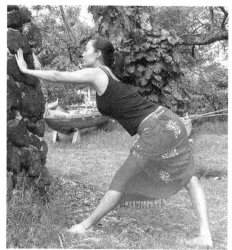

Alternative, both sides of legs and hips stretch.

Adductor Magnus

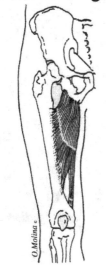

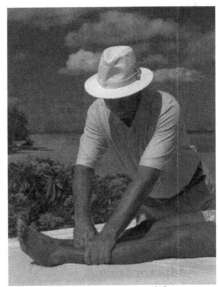

Adductor Magnus Muscle　　　　　**The Test for Adductors**

Origin: Edge of the entire ramus of the pubis and the ischium, as well as the tuberosity of the ischium outer and inferior.

Insertion: The whole length of the linea aspera and the inner condyloid ridge.

Action: Adduction of the thigh at the hip. Outward rotation with adduction.

Palpation: Medial posterior surface of the thigh. Horseback riding, gripping with the legs. Not a very commonly used muscle group. Need to do some specific exercises, which can help strengthen weak knees especially the medial collateral ligament, and the knee stabilizer.

Lengthen: Any kind of split or abduction of the leg.

Strengthen: Adductor points, lying on side, lift bottom leg towards ceiling. Squeeze a therapy ball or basketball between legs. Leverage: Third class in adduction.

Massage: It's similar for all in the adductor group. Compression, longitudinal cleansing strokes, as well as cross fiber and DTF for injured sites or tendons.

Adductor Longus

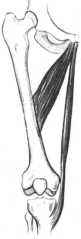

Adductor Longus

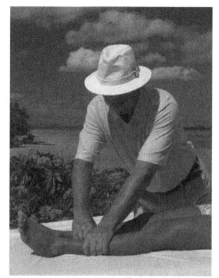

The Test

Origin: Front inferior ridge of the pubis, just below its crest.

Insertion: Middle third of the linea aspera on the medial ridge of the femur. The adductor brevis is the same except the insertion is more proximal on the upper fourth of the linea aspera of the femur.

Action: True adduction of the thigh at the hip, and also assists in flexion of the thigh at the hip. Horseback riding, gripping with the legs. Not a very commonly used muscle group. Need to do some specific exercises, which can help strengthen weak knees, especially the medial collateral ligament, and knee stabilizer as well.

Palpation: Medial posterior surface of the thigh.

Lengthen: Any kind of split or abduction of the leg.
Strengthen: Adductor points, lying on side, lift bottom leg towards ceiling. Squeeze a therapy ball or basketball.
Leverage: Third class in adduction.

Inner Thigh or Groin Pull

These groin pulls can be very serious, and can take a long time to heal. Most athletes at sometime or another have injured these adductor muscles. They pull your legs together and if you have spread them too far, as in reaching for the bag at first base, or just running too hard before you warmed up correctly, this injury often occurs. Racquetball and tennis come to mind, since many people rarely stretch enough when playing these sports. It can be a mild injury and only hurt when you push the body, or if you stretch too far. It can also be serious enough to hurt for years, especially with re-injury. Other injuries to this area can result from horseback riding too much when you are not used to it.

Test

Have the patient supine and have them hold their legs together tight. You stabilize one leg with one hand and pull at the ankle with the other. If this hurts you can find the area and know what it is. If it's not conclusive you may have them sit, cross legged with the knees up high, and then have them resist as you push both knees down with your hand.

RICE will help if you start right away. Never stretch a groin pull. DTF will help accelerate the healing as well, but you need to be very precise with the location of the lesion or it will not help much. Deep massage later will help increase circulation as well as deep cross fiber work.

Of course if that doesn't help an injection will increase the healing and also works well for chronic problems. Because of the location, for prevention of further injuries it's good to squeeze a ball with the knees to strengthen this group.

Gracilis

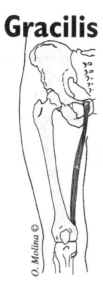

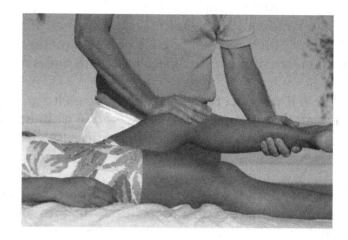

Gracilis Muscle   The test pull the leg out from ankle area stabilize knee.

Origin: The inner edge of the descending ramus of the pubis, most lateral.

Insertion: The anterior medial surface of the tibia below and inferior to the condyle.

Action: True adduction of the thigh at the hip, also assists in flexion of the thigh at the knee. Inward rotation as well. Horseback riding, griping with the legs. Not a very commonly used muscle group. Need to do some specific exercises, which can help strengthen weak knees, especially the medial collateral ligament, and knee stabilizer as well.

Palpation: Medial inside surface of the thigh.

Lengthen: Any kind of split or abduction of the leg.
Strengthen: Adductor points, lying on side lift bottom leg towards ceiling. Squeeze a therapy ball or basketball.
Leverage: Third class in adduction.

Biceps Femoris

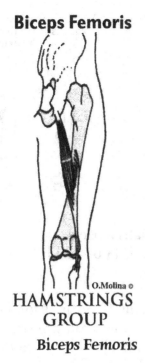

O.Molina ©

**HAMSTRINGS
GROUP**

Biceps Femoris

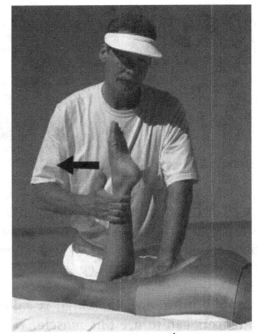

Hamstring Test

Origin: The inferior aspect of the ischial tuberosity, lower half of the linea aspera and the outer condyloid ridge.

Insertion: The lateral condyle of the tibia and the lateral head of the fibula.

Action: Extension of the thigh at the hip, one of the three in the hamstring group. Flexion of the leg at the knee, as well as outward rotation of the femur. (External Rotation) Works with the gluteus maximus in running, jumping, etc.

Strengthen: By squats, lunges, deep knee bends, as they work in extension of the hip, but weights are much more effective for this particular group

Lengthening: This muscle group is critical for effective running as well as for less stress on the low back. Massage: see hamstring group.

Rectus Femoris

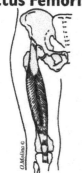

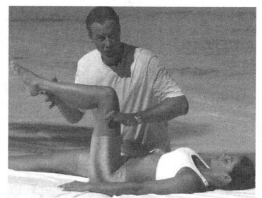

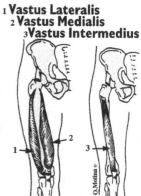

1 **Vastus Lateralis**
2 **Vastus Medialis**
3 **Vastus Intermedius**

Quadriceps test: push down on knee,

Rectus femoris (Quad 1)

Vastus Intermedius muscle (2)

The Quadriceps Muscle and Upper Leg

Vastus Medialis muscle (3)

Vastus lateralis (4 of Quads)

The muscle usually injured in the thigh is called the rectus femoris. Runners, football players, and dancers can injure this muscle. This muscle is the main hip flexor; in other words, it helps you lift the knee. The rest of the quads (see knee) only extend the leg at the knee (straighten the leg). The higher it hurts, the more likely you injured the tendon. If the pain is down on the middle of the leg, you may have some micro-tears in the muscle tissue. This tissue can be injured in contact sports (football, rugby or soccer). It can also be injured in a slip or fall. Of course, over use in running can injure this muscle, and it can also be overstretched by novice runners pulling too hard on their ankles, stretching it cold.

Test

As above, two tests can be done for the quads. First, if the injury is high, with the patient sitting have them try and lift their knee towards the ceiling as you resist, holding down their thigh (hip flexors). Next have them lay supine, bend the knee at the hip holding the leg in a 90% and then stabilize the knee while the other hand pushes down on the ankle. This will set off the pain in the tissue that is injured.

Treatment

This injury responds well to MICE. Movement with the ice bag would consist of slight extensions and contractions of the leg while sitting. This could last four to six weeks if the injury is severe. Of course, DTF is great for this muscle especially on the muscle itself. If the tendon is injured DTF is very painful, so be careful. You may need to hang the leg off the table to get a good stretch on it because it is a deep tendon. Deep tissue massage should never be done directly on the lesion, as you will separate the tear further. However, all around the area it is great to use since it increases circulation and aids in reducing the edema.

For a serious tear you may need to see a doctor. A corticosteroid injection to the ligament can work wonders and can reduce unwanted scar tissue. Remember, you need to bench the athlete after these injections.

Origin: The outer surface of the femur below the greater trochanter and the upper half of the linea aspera on the femur. All the quadriceps muscles origin on the femur. The only hip flexor of this group is the rectus femoris.

Insertion: The outer half of the superior border of the patella and the patellar ligament on the tibial tuberosity.

Action: Extension of the leg at the knee, on the lateral middle side of the thigh.

Strengthen: Squats, leg work like jumping, running, lunges, weight training, leg extensions and squat rack.

Lengthen: pulling the heels to the buttocks, kneeling and bending the body backwards. Be careful to keep the knees straight, don't bow out the feet or it will stress the knee ligaments.

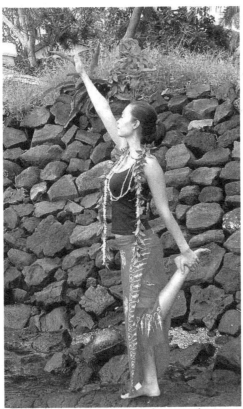

Easy standing quad stretch...

Popliteus

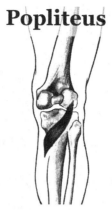

Popliteus Muscle

Origin: Posterior surface of the later (outer) condyle of the femur

Insertion: Upper posterior medial surface of the tibia.

Action: Flexion of the leg at the knee. Works with the quadriceps in stabilizing the knee and in action with the hamstrings in walking and running.

Strengthen: Leg curls on machines or squats and lunges.

Massage: Hard to palpate except for part of the origin and insertion. Apply DTF and some circular massage as well.

.

CHAPTER TWENTY NINE
The Lower Legs

Gastrocnemius

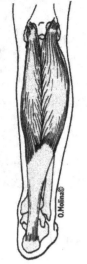

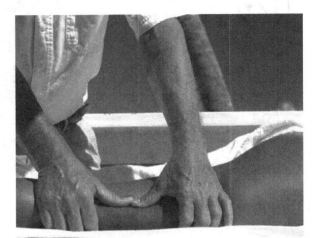

The Gastrocnemius Muscle (calves) Picture of cross fiber on Gastrocnemius origin

Origin: The posterior surfaces of the two condyles of the femur, posterior aspect.

Insertion: The posterior surface of the calcaneus at the heel.

Action: The main function is plantar flexion of the foot, flexion of the leg at the knee.

Strengthen: Calf raises, pushing off on toes on a block, lowering heels below the balls of the feet.

Lengthen: Bringing toes up, or dorsiflexion. Leaning against the wall, etc.

Massage: Always start with compression on big muscles. Deep work on this muscle is critical. Sometimes it can cause cramps, so be careful. The middle stroke is good, after on either side of the center. Then circles around the main head of the muscle up medial, down lateral side. Cross fiber strokes on this muscle are very effective.

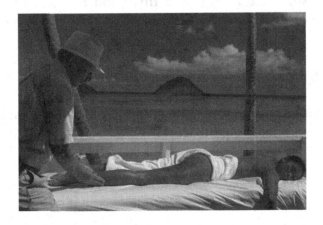

Soleus

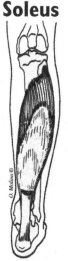

The Soleus Muscle

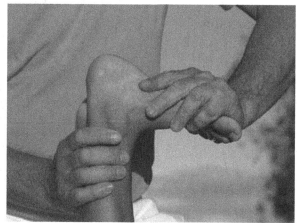

Test: have patient push off your hand

Origin: The upper two-thirds of the posterior surface of the tibia and the fibula.

Insertion: The posterior surface of the calcaneus.

Action: Plantar flexion of the foot.

Strength: Pushing off with the toes, plantar flexion along with the gastrocnemius. Squats, running, jumping, hopping, etc.

Lengthen: Pointing toes up towards the tibia, dorsal flexion.

Massage: Same as gastrocnemius, it's much deeper so you have to work deep. Compression massage is especially helpful for this muscle.

Tibialis Anterior

Origin: Upper two-thirds of the outer surface of the tibia.

Insertion: Inner surface of the medial cuneiform and the first metatarsal bones.

Action: Dorsi flexion, some adduction and inversion of the foot. Works harder when standing on the outside of the foot, or in skating. This is often the muscle that suffers shin splints.

Palpation: Just lateral to the tibia bone, antagonist to the plantar flexors.

Strengthen: Working out on tiptoes, opposite action from calf raises, the negative will work these muscles. To lengthen, same as quadriceps.

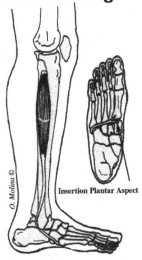
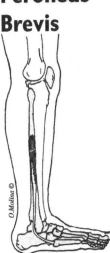
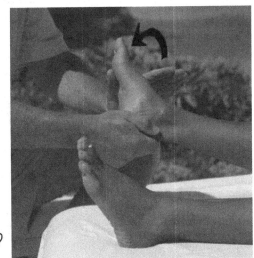

Peroneus Longus   **Peroneus Brevis**

Insertion Plantar Aspect

Peroneus Longus
& Peroneus Brevis

Test: push food medially supporting the heel.

Origin: Head of the fibula and the upper two-thirds of the surface of the lateral fibular ridge.

Insertion: Under surfaces (plantar side) of the medial cuneiform and the first metatarsal.

Action: Major plantar flexion with some eversion of the foot. (Turning out) Works with the anterior tibialis, its antagonist, in running and pushing off the foot.
Same as above. See peroneal tendonitis.

Flexor Hallucis Longus

Origin: The lower two-thirds of the posterior surface of the fibula.

Insertion: The base of the distal phalanx of the large toe, plantar surface.

Action: Plantar flexion and some inversion (foot inward).

See massage, strengthening, and lengthening for the flexors of the lower leg.

Flexor Digitorum Longus Muscle

Origin: The lower two-thirds of the posterior surface of the tibia.

Insertion: Plantar base of the distal phalanx of each of the four outer toes.

Action: Plantar flexion and inversion of the foot, works with gastrocnemius, and the soleus.

235

Tibialis Posterior

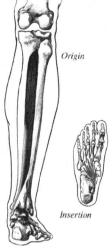

Origin

Insertion

Tibialis Posterior Muscle

Origin: Posterior surface of the upper half of the interosseous membrane and adjacent surfaces of the tibia and fibula.

Insertion: The lower plantar section of the navicular and the cuneiform bones and the base of the second, third, fourth and fifth metatarsal bones.

For action, strengthening, lengthening, and massage see flexors of the lower leg.

Flexor Digitorum Longus Muscle

Origin: Lower two-thirds of the posterior surface of the tibia.

Insertion: The base plantar side, of the distal phalanx of each of the front outer toes.

For action, strengthening, lengthening and massage see flexors of the lower leg.

Extensors of the Lower Leg
Extensor Digitorim Longus

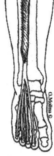

Extensor Digitorum Longus (extends the toes)

Origin: Outer condyle of the tibia, head of the fibula and the whole ridge of the upper two-thirds of the anterior surface of the fibula.

Insertion: The dorsal (top) of the medial and distal phalanges of the four outer toes.

Action: Dorsal flexion, some eversion of the foot (turn outward) and toe extension. Also stabilizes and works with the plantar flexors.

Strengthening: Only on negative calf raises, used mostly to balance the lower leg.

Lengthening and massage, same as above.

Extensor Hallucis Longus

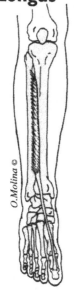

O.Molina ©

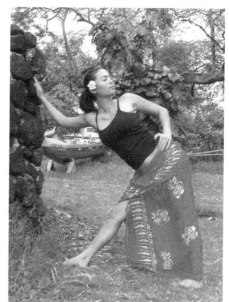

Extensor Hallucis Longus   A good all around stretch for the hips, legs, and back.

Origin: The middle two-thirds of the inner surface of the front of the fibula.

Insertion: The top of the distal phalanx of the great toe.

Action extension of the large toe aids in dorsi-flexion of the foot.

For action, strengthening, lengthening and massage see all the extensors of the lower leg.

CHAPTER THIRTY
The Knee Joint

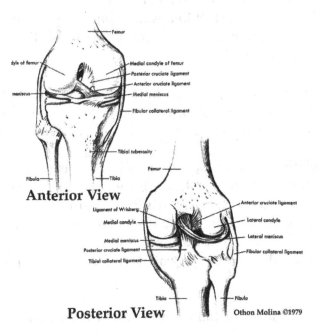

Anterior View

Posterior View

Othon Molina ©1979

The knee is the biggest joint in the body, and prone to injury in most athletic sports. The reason is because it only moves forward and backward, flexion and extension, so consequently, if there is any side to side stress on it, it will get hurt. I'm sure if you go to a football game, basketball game or even in a baseball game, someone hurts his or her knee.

Whenever someone gets hit like in football, it's the knee. Whenever you twist too fast, as in basketball, it's the knee, and the same for most other intense, fast cutting sports.

There are many injuries to the knee that come from just running. I believe that if your hips are out of alignment, your knee suffers from improper mechanical functioning, and you will eventually get some sort of pain in the knee. The jogging revolution has started many knee problems; I can't tell you how many patients come in with some sort of knee problem. There are over twenty potential knee injuries. If a patient comes in and can point right to the problem, it's not too difficult to figure out what it is, as long as you can do a resistance test and find the tendon, muscle or ligament. Torn cartilage is another tricky problem, as is bursitis or chondromalacia.

The knee is made up of the femur, the tibia, the fibula, and the patella, or kneecap. This floating bone is woven into the rectus femoris tendon (quadriceps muscle). It's a tendon that functions like a ligament originates at the hip and inserts at the tibia. The other major muscle groups are the hamstrings (see for a more detailed description). The knee is also held together with lots of ligaments. The major ligaments are the medial collateral (inside) and the lateral collateral ligaments (outside).

Then a common football or skiing injury is to the anterior cruciate ligament: This ligament is in the center of your knee, it holds the knee joint together with the posterior cruciate. They cross in the middle from the femur to the tibia.

The other ligaments in the knee, less frequently injured, are the medial coronary ligament and lateral coronary ligament. They hold the cartilage in place, the meniscus cartilage that acts as the shock absorber in the joint. It keeps the bones from rubbing against each other. Wearing away of any of this material can cause arthritis of the knee sometimes called chondromalacia, or other problems.

Fortunately, with state-of-the-art surgery, now athletes, after a properly done cruciate repair or reconstruction, can return to sports within the year. It used to end most athletes' careers. The anterior cruciate ligament is the most commonly injured ligament in the knee.

The ligaments have a relatively poor vascular supply and it is virtually impossible to heal a complete tear. Injuries of the ligament produce bleeding into the knee, which is the reason why you get a swollen knee after a rupture. Just like a muscle tear, the swelling represents blood in the joint. Once torn, the knee usually becomes unstable and can cause other injuries to the cartilage. The patients who remain in sports have a 75% chance of further damage to one or more of the important cartilage structures within the joint, and the potential for arthritis.

Prevention and protection against ligament injury and for an early return to athletics after ligament surgery are both achieved by strengthening the muscles around the knee. These muscles that act as shock absorbers and joint stabilizers need to be strengthened. Specifically, hamstring strength protects the tibia from the anterior translocation (from going too forward) that can rupture the cruciate. Often we see that the quadriceps are twice as strong as the hamstring group. So it's important to focus on the hamstrings to stabilize the knee joint. If the hamstrings are weak the knee goes into hypertension, thus creating the situation for injury.

When the skier "catches an edge" or in the cutting sports if you take a sharp turn, the stability is often dependent on the quadriceps and hamstring power for balance. It's a potential problem when you are on one ski and attempting to rein in the wayward leg. If the quadriceps muscles are weak, the leg wobbles under the unexpected load and twists as the skier or athlete falls, and "pop," you tear the cruciate. I have personally experienced this skiing in Canada, Of course, contact injuries to the knee will often tear the cruciate, for example in football when someone hits your knee and it bends backwards. I had the fortune of healing my cruriate tear, with herbs, acupuncture, massage and then strengthening at the right time. I have no problem with the knee. It takes a great amount of knowledge and dedication to heal something as severe, but it can be done.

The knee also has many bursars and these fluid sacks also get injured, especially the one under the kneecap. This kind of pain may feel like a dull ache, and of course, often knee injuries can actually cause damage to several tissues as well as the structures of the knee. Careful examination is necessary.

Pain in the Front of the Knee

Patellar tendonitis is one of the most common over-use syndromes dealing with the knee joint. Many runners get this, in fact, they often call it "runners knee." Like the Achilles tendonitis, it's a problem to diagnose because the pain comes and goes. It seems to hurt during running and intense walking. It can hurt to climb stairs. It only hurts all the time when it's in the acute phase. Then it seems to get better if you rest it for a few days. Then, of course, if you run again it hurts again. It can hurt all around the patella. Although it is actually a tear or a strain of the patellar tendon, doing the test can tell for certain.

Causes for Injury

The most common cause for injury in this tendon is not warming up and stretching the quads properly. Another reason, in my opinion, is poor alignment of the hips and so the knees take unusual stress when running. Often it is because the muscles are too tight and pull to heavily on the tendon. Also, check the fit of the running shoes and check the foot for flat feet or poor arch support. Orthodics may be needed in the long term correction of this condition.

The Muscles of the Knee

The quads are actually four major muscles: the rectus femoris, the vastus lateralis, the vastus medialis and the vastus Intermedius. On the front of the leg also attaching on the knee are the fascia lata, the sartorius, and the adductor groups.

On the posterior side of the knee as we said are the hamstrings. This muscle group is actually the biceps femoris, the vastus lateralis, the semitendinosis, the semimembranosis, the gracilis, the popliteus, and the plantaris. Below the knee in the rear are also the calf muscles or the gastrocnemius, the soleus, the plantaris, and the peroneus. See the specific muscles for more detail on testing and action of these muscles.

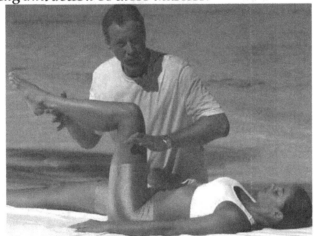

Testing of the Rectus Femoris for Patellar Tendonitis

Because this muscle is so strong and the pain may be defused it's best to test the muscle after it has been worked. When it's exhausted it will be easier to test for the problem. With the patient supine, bend the knee at the hip and hold the knee at a 90 degree angle.

Press hard on the tibia while stabilizing the knee with the other hand. If the tendon is injured this will set off the pain, and you will be able to locate it by palpation. Often you may not get a very specific pain site so you may need to have them run up and down some stairs or do some deep knee bends (careful with this as this may hurt too much). This can often get confused with chondromalacia or bursitis of the knee; however, these are usually felt deeper in the knee joint.

Treatment

RICE is the recommended treatment for this condition and, of course, rest and stop running. Using an ice bag with gentle movement is very helpful. It's a variation of RICE which I call MICE (Movement, Ice, Compression and Elevation). The movement will allow the body to heal without creating too much scar tissue. After two to three weeks of rest you may start with easy activities. If it's not better after four weeks you should see a doctor.

Of course, DTF is very effective for this injury, but it can hurt so you have to go easy. Also during the acute phase you could friction with the ice cube.

If it's an old injury that has acted up due to unusual activity, such as training for a marathon in your forties, sometimes a well-placed injection of some corticosteroid is beneficial. Of course, with this must come rest. Sometimes one or two injections are all it takes to turn it around.

The other factor is if it's poor foot stability that contributes to this condition it may take orthodics for correcting the problem.

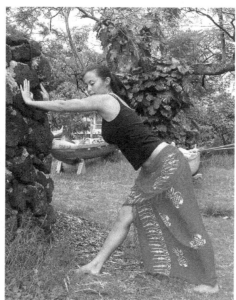

Quadriceps stretch standing (left) the hurdler stretch also works the key is to keep the knee straight as well as the foot do not twist it out. Also an all around leg and hip stretch.

The Cruciate Ligament Injury

This ligament is a broad, thick cord the size of a person's index finger. It has long collagen strands woven in a fashion that permits forces of up to 500 pounds to be exerted on it before it rips. If that occurs it is a serious injury and very common in football or skiing. Of course, when hit from the front the knee bends backwards. It can also be a long term over-use type of injury where it slowly comes on and then is set off by an unusual event.

Pain deep in the knee joint is a common complaint. It's hard to locate the pain because it's so deep in the joint. One sign of this injury is when the person cannot walk downhill because they feel that their knee joint is going to give out. Walking stairs is also difficult as the joint is less stable. The ligament is crucial for guiding the tibia in a normal path along the end of the femur and maintaining the joint stability.

It can also be torn in a quick motion such as a fall, or running in a fast sprint. This is more unusual but it does happen. Sometimes before the drawer test I may just check with the following test, moving the femur opposite the tibia (see below).

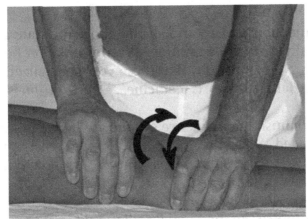

Move back and forth against each other. (TOP)

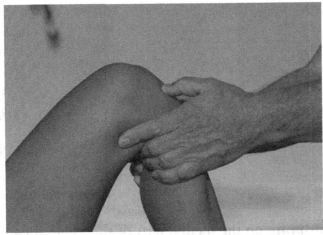

The Drawer Test

These tests should only be done if the pain is mild, as you may have just strained the ligament. If the pain is severe and you can hardly bend your knee, see a doctor.

The test for this injury is called the drawer test. The patient lies supine on the table and bends the knee at the hip, resting the foot on the table. The therapist then pushes at the tibia and forces the tibia posterior. Any play in this joint during this push indicates a weak or partially torn cruciate ligament. It will hurt at times, yet other times you don't get the pain that may be felt during walking. This pain can be a dull ache and not sharp as with other ligament injuries. If it hurts in the back part of the knee it could be a posterior cruciate injury. Keeping the knee in the same position, grasp behind the knee while sitting on their foot to stabilize it, and then pull forward and check for motion or pain.

Treatment

Treatment for this injury is MICE (ice will always help) but because the tissue is so deep in the knee there is really no massage that can be done other than working on all the peripheral muscles in the leg. Prevention of this injury is better and less painful for the athletes that do the sports where this injury is common (football, skiing, rugby, track, basketball, and baseball). Building up the knee joint is imperative, not only by building up the muscles but you can also build up the ligaments, they just take much longer. (See building the base.)

I have also heard that injections in this area during the acute state are able to increase the healing if it's just partially torn. They even use proliferants that help create scar tissue to help support this injury. Note, however, that these very specialized treatments need to be done by a doctor that specializes in sports medicine, as the location is very difficult to reach.

Specific exercises can diminish the incidence of cruciate ligament injury. Most often if it is torn badly surgery is needed. Nowadays, our surgical approaches can promptly correct this injury permitting an early return to sports. This injury is serious and usually requires surgical repair or reconstruction.

Injuries to the Medial Collateral Ligament

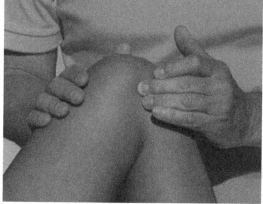

Palpate Medial Ligament

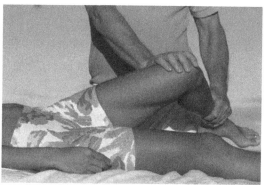

Test medial ligaments

This is a very common ligament sprain on the medial part of the knee. It can come and go and gets irritated with activity in its mild form. If it is more severe it can knock you down, and it will swell up and hurt a lot. After a few weeks the pain is more concentrated in the points in the picture above. The pain may come and go and can be confusing.

If it came on suddenly, once again I blame misalignment of the pelvis, especially if there is knock-knees. Too much tension in the fascia lata can also be a factor. Sometimes old injuries that have formed improper scar tissue hold the ligament too tight and will create further injuries. Then you let it heal, and the cycle starts all over again.

The test for the medial collateral is to have the patient supine and bend their leg medially. The therapist puts pressure on the medial side of the knee, trying to open the two bones. This causes the ligament to stretch and causes the pain, if the tissue is injured.

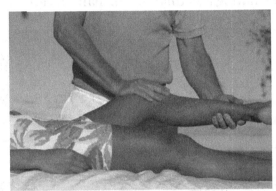

The test for the lateral collateral ligament.

The test for the lateral collateral ligament is the opposite: Your hand is placed on the medial part of the knee joint and the pressure is lateral (overstretching the ligaments will hurt laterally.) This injury is less frequent and for some reason it heals faster than the medial.

MICE is great, the movement with the ice bag keeps scar tissue from forming between the ligament and the bones. DTF done every other day for at least four weeks will help heal and prevent the improperly formed scar tissue. If it's old and chronic, DTF will be painful but will help make a subtler tissue. Manipulations to increase ROM may be necessary to pull the old scar tissue off the bone. Professionals trained in sports medicine or sports massage must do these treatments.

Some clinics use diathermy and ultrasound to aid in healing. My experience shows these to be less effective than DTF.

Sometimes injections can stop the inflammation and pain. This will allow the body to increase healing. The corticosteroid will reduce inflammation and the proliferants will help tighten loose and overstretched ligaments. If the tear is bad enough sometimes a cast is put on the leg, but these days this is not often done because severe scar tissue can form and freeze up the knee joint. Surgery is the other treatment when the ligament is completely torn. This should be done as soon as possible with DTF, deep massage, and manipulations used in the rehab period.

Pain in the Tensor Fascia Lata, Outside of the Knee

This again is a very common injury for runners, especially distance runners and athletes that do a lot of fast cutting such as in football, rugby, basketball, and soccer. With a tear or a strain on this tendon, the pain is felt just above and to the outside of the knee, at the insertion of the fascia lata. It's actually all fascia down at this point since the muscle is short up at the hip. It's an over-use type of injury. Once again the pain comes on with heavy activity and then feels better at night. It does not get swollen very often so you go train again and it hurts again, each time taking less time for the pain to return.

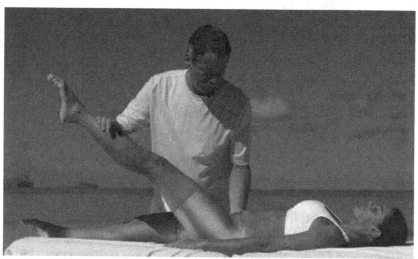

Test

To test this tendon have the patient supine, holding the leg up for the fascia lata test. Exert pressure medially on the lateral part of the tibia. If this hurts in the spot suspected, palpate for the lesion.

Treatment

RICE of course, with some movement, flexing and extending the knee with the ice bag. In addition to DTF, massage is very effective for this injury; in fact, prevention of this injury by deep massage and friction on the tendons may help most runners. I have always found this fascia is very tight in most people. Once again, prevention is less painful.

A well placed injection may also help if the injury is more severe. However, taking the athlete out of training is imperative. I used to have them swim with a floater between their legs to keep up cardiovascular fitness during the recovery. Easy bike workouts can be done within three to four weeks so that scar tissue does not bind up the knee joint. Running should only be resumed after there is no pain in doing that activity.

Hamstring Injury or Pain on the Inside of the Knee

These are common sprinter injuries as well as from fast cutting sports. You may feel pain on the back of the knee (hamstring tendon) or sometimes on the front below the knee joint (hamstrings insertion). The hamstring group is composed of three muscles and they all originate from one tendon at the ischial tuberosity, or our sit bones. They then split up and some go on the outside of the knee and some on the inside of the knee. They then insert at the lateral and medial condyle of the tibia. Part of the biceps femoris inserts on part of the head of the fibula as well. This is a common site for injury as well. (See peroneus test)

Pain here is also due to over use or pushing yourself beyond your capabilities. It often hurts worse later because as the tendon cools, pain returns.

This is an injury due to lack of flexibility. Many runners have very tight hamstrings. Sometimes it's from lack of warm up and so the tight muscle tears when pushed.

Stretching is what you don't want to do to any tendon or muscle when injured. So often I have treated people that keep that injury going because someone stretching tells them it will make it better. As I said early on, the other cause is from muscles that are out of balance. Usually the quadriceps are twice as strong as the hamstrings making this joint unstable; they then have to do more work and are prone to injury. The ratio should be about 60% quads and 40% hamstrings. I always work my hamstrings twice what I work the quads. We use the quads much more frequently as in walking, moving to a standing position, and walking up stairs. We use the hamstrings much less as they are designed to bend the knee and raising our heel to our buttocks.

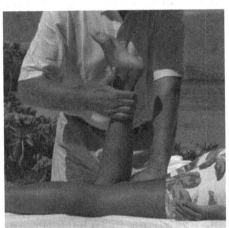

To Test the Hamstrings

Place the patient prone; bend the leg at the knee in a 90 degree angle. Stabilize the leg at the hamstrings and pull down holding while the ankle. You will note pain either medially or laterally. Palpate for the injury and follow standard treatment for a tendon or muscle injury.

Treatment

MICE (movement is important for this injury as you don't want improperly formed scar tissue). Extend and flex the knee with the ice bag on it two or three times a day, with five to ten sets of extensions minimally. DO NOT STRETCH during the acute phase and don't run for four to five weeks. DTF massage is great for this, making sure the tendon is stretched to just about 80% of its full length, and friction the sore spot. Using ice for the friction massage should be done for forty-eight hours. Then you can friction without ice every other day. Be careful not to create more irritation, as it will then take longer to heal. If the athlete wants to workout, have them swim and kick very gently.

If that hurts have them use a floater between the legs and not kick at all for two weeks. The best way to start back on training would be to use a bike until there is no pain with that activity. Then and only then can they resume running but gently. If pain occurs during running, it's back to the bike. The area most common for this injury is at the insertion points of the tendons; in fact, just rub any runner there and they will have some pain. Prevention of this injury can be done with lots of good stretching and DTF at the origin and insertion of the muscles.

Deep massage will help if it's not done right on the injured tendon. It can reduce the pull on the rest of the leg and hips. Working on the gluteus muscles will reduce tension on the knee joint as well as the whole leg area.

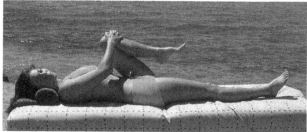

An easy stretch and lengthen technique for the hamstrings.

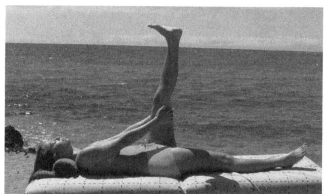

A more advanced stretch for the hamstring, keep back flat and tighten abdominal muscles

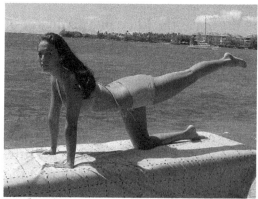

Good strengthening exercise for hamstrings and gluteals.

Chondromalacia or Pain under the Kneecap

This is like sciatica; Lots of people think that they have this condition when it's actually something else since it's not that common. The pain is a dull ache like bursitis and when severe it can hurt the whole knee area. It usually happens in both knees as it's a condition where the lubrication of the knee is poor and the cartilage surrounding the patella gets worn down.

The bones then start to rub together (they can actually create a grinding sound) and patients say their knees creek all the time when they walk. Just sitting can make the knees hurt. Walking up or down stairs will also hurt, and forget about kneeling down, the pain can get severe.

Once again misalignment of the body is one of the causes, as is sometimes a nutritional deficiency. If you have flat feet your more likely to pronate (turn in, see feet section) the feet. This puts more stress and straining on the knee joint, and stress like this can cause it to wear it down.

Test

The test for this condition is no fun and can really hurt, so be careful. The patient is sitting with the legs extended. Place your hand on the patella and push down on it and move it from side to side. If you hear a grinding sound or it feels like there is gravel in the knee joint, it may be chondromalacia. It may also hurt without the sound if there is bursitis, so check for that and for patellar tendonitis as well.

Treatment

There's not much you can do with massage other than prevention of the stress. Then again you can reduce the stress and pain in the other muscle groups that are in reaction to the pain. Ice may help temporarily but not for the long term. Anti-inflammatory drugs can reduce some of the swelling but don't really produce a cure. Exercises don't really help, nor do corticosteroid injections, they are all temporary. Proliferant injections can help when the condition is not too severe, as it can stabilize the joint causing less stress.

Nutritional supplements such as glucosamine, or high doses of bromelain (pineapple enzyme) help; however, neither have been medically proven. It is a mysterious problem. The best thing to do is to avoid the activities that cause the pain. I have heard of some treatments in Europe where they inject a jelly type substance into the joint to help lubricate better. It's called Dimethylpolysiloxane, not DMSO. (Benjamin)

Injury to Meniscus Cartilage

Torn cartilage is a common injury as well in most sports. It happens a lot in football, basketball, and with some dancers and gymnasts. This can come from a sudden twist, as well as long term abuse. These tears can hurt deep in the knee so the pain can be confused with other injuries. What makes this easy to figure out is the patient will say "I was walking or running and my knee gave out" or "the knee locked up." Sometimes the piece of cartilage gets in the way of the two bones and gets pinched. This feels like someone has stuck a knife in your knee (I have had several of these injuries). The knee feels very unstable similar to the anterior cruciate injury but it locks or gives you a very sharp pain for no reason in easy movements. Sometimes just rolling over in bed can cause the patient to want to jump out of their skin.

First of all, if you suspect a cartilage tear send them to a doctor. There are several tests, all of which can tear the cartilage worse if you are not careful. Usually with the symptoms mentioned above, you will more than likely not get this test. It involves the therapist holding your knee with one hand and your ankle with the other. Then you twist the knee medially and laterally. This produces the sharp pain in the deep part of the knee joint. (Same as above for medial and lateral meniscus).

Most often you will require an arthrogram, which is an x-ray with an injection of dye into the knee. The dye allows you to see the tear. Often it is necessary to get an MRI (magnetic resonance imaging). This system works by a type of sonar with magnetic properties and creates images similar to x-rays; however, it does show soft tissue injuries. This allows the doctor to really see the tear and injury to the cartilage.

Sometimes injury to the **medial coronary ligament** gets confused with a meniscus tear, or often both are present, **lateral coronary ligament**

The way to tell the difference is that the test for these two ligaments is slightly different. For the medial coronary ligament: Place the patient supine and bend the knee. Then you stabilize the knee joint with one hand more lateral to the knee and you place some torque on the foot pushing laterally. This puts stress on the medial coronary ligament, causing the pain medially. This injury responds well to DTF and the treatment described below.

To test the lateral coronary ligament you place the bent leg in the same position and you push on the lateral side of the foot moving medial. This stresses the lateral side of this ligament. Following the treatment is similar, except that for DTF you can't reach all the parts of this ligament except for the anterior part, as the rest is deep in the knee cavity.

Treatment

Initially RICE can help heal this injury if it's minor. However, if it locks up on you to the degree that it swells severely and causes pain for weeks, see a doctor.

Massage does nothing for this condition once it's happened. There are some manipulations of the knee joint that may help to place the meniscus back in alignment, but if it's torn it will just come out again.

Injections of corticosteroid can help heal the area; however, you must really rest after this injection. Then there are the proliferants (a mixture of lydocain and dextrose) that create scar tissue, which can allow the injury some support and the healing can begin.

These are all for minor injuries but once there is a severe tear, arthroscopic surgery may be required. They go in and trim off the piece of cartilage. Since cartilage has very little blood flow, they heal very slowly and often massage and other health treatments can accelerate the recovery. Some people just live without the surgery and don't have too many problems, but this is one time that I recommend surgery if it bugs you. It is an easy operation when done by a good doctor and the results are good.

Bursitis or Water on the Knee

This condition can come from an injury or develop gradually. This again can often be due to misalignment of the knee joint, of the foot, or of the hip. The swelling is the body's mechanism to heal and immobilize an area to prevent further injury.

Again, it can hurt to bend the knee or to kneel down. The tests are by kneeling and putting extreme pressure on the patella. The therapist may have the patient sit with the legs extended. Then place your thumb just distal to the patella and press down. This should hurt if the patient has a hard time fully extending the knee and if there is noticeable swelling, it could be very severe. Just as in the shoulder, manipulations or DTF massage will not help, if anything they can make it worse. Have the patient see a doctor. The best way to start the healing cycle is with an injection of corticosteroid, which reduces the inflammation better than anything else. It may take several injections and you should see improvement right away.

As prevention for the future, look at the posture and do an extensive orthopedic and kinesiological examination to determine potential factors.

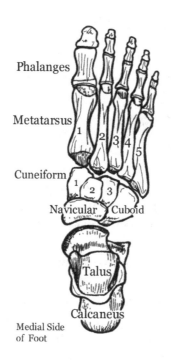

Phalanges

Metatarsus

Cuneiform

Navicular   Cuboid

Talus

Calcaneus

Medial Side
of Foot

CHAPTER THIRTY ONE
The Foot and Ankle

Your feet are the foundation for your body; at least, they are at the bottom of your whole structure. They are often a cause of many other problems. To me, the feet are very important and I spend a lot of time working on them, especially with athletes and dancers. They are the ones that will put greater demands on the whole bottom part of the body and all the way up to the low back. We know that feet can cause other problems, i.e., flat feet, low leg and lower back problems. We also must understand that when your body is out of alignment, your feet need to reflect that weight re-distribution. Consequently, when you work on alignment for the body you need to align the feet as well. By giving the bones in the feet some new patterns once you do that it can adapt to the new hip alignment. In fact, the whole body is connected, so if you want to change anything you need to work on every joint in the body as well.

The bones of the feet are the calcaneus; the talus; the navicular; the cuboid; three cuneiform bones; five metatarsals, and phalanges. About 22 bones and 26 joints make up the foot structure.

The feet are made to take a tremendous amount of pressure; they were designed to take up to 2500 pounds per square inch of torque. (I don't know how they measured this but that's what we are told.) The reason there are so many bones in the foot is so it can displace the pressure exerted on them. These many joints and surfaces give them strength as well as flexibility. Many people have foot problems, mainly because our feet weren't meant to be strapped into non-flexible shoes.

When you don't allow feet the full movement, the muscles do not get worked properly, and you won't strengthen the ligaments by normal, progressive resistance training. The muscles and ligaments get stiff and weak because of the rigid soles. Part of training athletes needs to incorporate more barefoot running in the sand and on uneven surfaces. Another big factor in preventing feet and ankle injuries is specificity in training: If you are going to take sharp turns, make quick stops, and use explosive movements you must build up the ligaments, muscles, and connective tissues to take on that load. You can actually even build the bones and make them stronger.

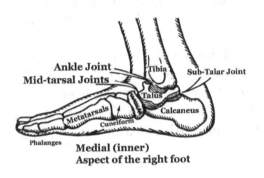

Medial (inner)
Aspect of the right foot

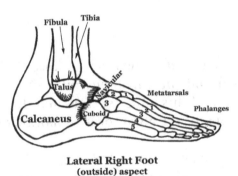

Lateral Right Foot
(outside) aspect

The Ankle

The ankle is also very strong and is formed from two of the leg bones, the tibia, which is the larger bone, and the fibula on the lateral side, which is smaller. These two bones articulate at the ankle as well as proximal at the knee.

The close approximation of these two bones makes and shapes the ankle joint. These two bones make up the "ankle mortise" (like a carpenter's mortise and tendon joint in furniture making) and they envelop the talus called the "internal ankle bone." The prominence of the distal (far) end of the tibia makes the medial malleolus, or the inside ankle bone, while the bulge of the distal (far) end of the fibula makes the prominence called the lateral malleolus, or outside ankle bone.

The talus is surrounded on three sides by these bones of the leg because of the mortise joint configuration. So any rotation (twisting inward or outward) on the long axis of the leg causes the talus and leg to move in unison as one unit.

Most internal (inward) rotation that causes the leg and kneecap to face more toward the middle of the body also causes the talus to face more toward the middle of the body.

External (or outward) rotation would cause the leg and kneecap as well as the talus to face away from the middle of the body.

It's not really a motion at the ankle joint but more of a change in the actual alignment of the ankle due to a rotation of the superstructure described above (at the leg, the tibia, and fibula). On the other hand, the talus has not moved relative to the leg bones above. The only motion of the ankle is true plantar flexion (toes go down), and dorsiflexion (toes go up), which are the downward and upward parts of the movement of walking.

With ankle-type joint motion there is more of a change in the relationship of the upper leg bones (tibia and fibula) to the talus. In the walking gait, the ankle joint's function is to permit the forward movement of the body. It moves over the planted or the stable part of the foot. The strengthening of this area is best done by running in the sand or by walking with an intense gait, with an exaggerated push off and with wide stepping. (See Percy Curitty's work.)

The Subtalar Joint
(Or below the talus bone)

This is an extremely complicated joint known as "the lower ankle joint" and it is formed by the talus superior (see above) and the calcaneus inferior, or the heel bone (see below). Consequently, the configuration of this joint's surface and the angles of these surfaces make the motion not as purely and simply a straight forward motion of up and down.

Rather, this motion actually occurs in three different directions simultaneously. This motion is "pronation and suppination," in other words, the joint moves inwards or outwards. When this joint is neither "pronated" nor "suppinated" it is said to be "in the neutral position."

Flat feet are a different level of pronation. Duck feet (feet that are turned out) are a different level of suppination. Most common injuries to the ankle are in suppination. This is at the talo-fibular tendon, ligaments on the lateral side (outside of the ankle).

Too high an arch can give you pain in the heel or in the ball of the foot, and at times, weak anterior tibialis or posterior tibialis may also be involved. In weight bearing, whenever the leg internally (inwardly) rotates the subtalar joint pronates (outwardly), and whenever the leg externally (outwardly) rotates, the subtalar joint suppinates (inwardly). They work in opposing action.

As said earlier, suppination is associated with a well defined, higher arched foot while pronation is associated with a collapsed or flat foot.

The subtalar joint absorbs the torque through the foot. Similar to a universal joint in a car that changes the direction of rotation in the drive train and moves the wheels forward.

The subtalar joint takes rotation (medial or lateral) of the leg and converts this torque to forward motion within the foot (dorsiflexion and plantar flexion). The subtalar joint is also the main shock absorber for the foot so important for long distance runners who are prone to stress and injury.

This motion along with heel strike and slight pronation are the most efficient ways to absorb the shock from running. If this area is tight or out of alignment it can transfer the shock to the knee. It can also work its way up to the low back and or to the pelvis.

Because of the subtalar joint motion, we can walk on uneven surfaces, and twist and bend our ankles at the base of the leg. This is our stability joint, which supports all types of motion.

The Midtarsal Joint
(The joint in the middle)

This is more like two joints that function as one. The first part and superior is the talo-navicular joint where the talus bone meets the navicular (distal) bone. The motion of the foot is dependent on the motion between these two bones. This joint can get locked along with the foot in "the neutral position." The second part of this joint (inferior) is the calcaneus-cuboid joint where the calcaneus and the cuboid (distal) bones meet.

Pronation and suppination affect the working of this joint. Many runners suffer in this area, and often it takes some good manipulations to free up the locked up, mid tarsal joint. Poor arch support can injure this joint as well.

Lack of mobility here makes the foot a rigid structure, not only causing shock to the ankle joint itself, but also moving the shock up the leg to the knee, the trochanter, or the back.

Distal to this joint (furthest from the body) are the three cuneiform (or wedge shaped) bones and the five long metatarsal bones. The distal aspect of the five metatarsals forms what we commonly call the ball of the foot.

The first two metatarsals are the part of the big toe, which is often another source of injury occurring with running, or cutting sports, and sometimes causing injury on the plantar surface (bottom of foot) with some forms of plantar fasciatis. (See injuries to the foot.)

If the first metatarsal is blocked or has some scar tissue keeping it from absorbing shock, the stress or torque gets transferred to the second metatarsal. This can often cause the whole foot to stress and ache. If running is continued it leads to all kinds of injuries to the feet, as well as potential knee or back problems.

Malfunctions or Aberrations of the Foot

There are 22 bones and 26 joints in each foot, which is designed to take all the shock from walking and running as well as the stress from just standing. Did you ever stand all day at a new job? Your feet are killing you; we all know what that's like. Then after some time you get used to it. That's called building a base. Well, the other problem we have created for ourselves are stiff and poorly designed shoes. If you don't walk barefoot enough, you will not actively stretch and move all these little bones in your feet and they become even more rigid. You will certainly not strengthen those little, peripheral, support muscles in there, either. With more than 15 different tendons going through the ankle and feet, it's a complicated area to work with. This is why it's also a common area for injury.

Flat Feet

There are many types of foot problems, the most common being flat feet. There are many levels of flatness. The main problem is that you need that arch support and without it, it locks up the mid tarsal joint.

Some theorize that it's weakness in the anterior and posterior tibialis muscles, the Peroneus group, or even the flexor digitorum longus that cause the foot to have no arch. Either way, from faulty mechanics inherited or from weakness, this can be a problem for any runner. There are many theories why we have flat feet. There are many reasons why a foot will malfunction, and to give full explanations would need a great deal of detail and greater mechanical information following. The problem with rigidity or weakness causes problems.

High Arches

Normally high arches are not considered a problem. But if they are too high, just imagine: You don't have the full surface on the ground for support. This can create problems with the heel or the ball of the foot.

The foot is an extension or the foundation of the leg bones, so if you think of them as working together (and we should), the tibia is connected to the talus on the inside or medial area. The fibula is connected to the lateral or outside part of the talus. There are a lot of very strong ligaments here. When you have extremely high arches, it is thought that the support for these structures is not as efficient, and problems with the ligaments as well as with the fascia and muscles can arise.

Sources: This whole foot section came from some old manuscripts from the University of Hawaii. I could not find the writers names of this work and I would give them credit if I found them. Please let me know if you know them, as I had nothing as great as this for the feet. Thank you!

The Muscles of the Ankle and Foot

Coming into the ankle from the lateral side of the leg is the anterior tibialis, the peroneus longus, and brevis, the tendon of the extensor hallucis longus. More medially (on the inside of the leg), is the soleus, which is actually not just on the sole of the foot. It's also just to the medial (inside) of the tibia and the gastrocnemius both laterally, medially and rear. More on the posterior, it is one of the muscles most injured. Next to sprained ankles, the Achilles tendon is the second most injured muscle in the foot. It's the muscle that anchors the calf or gastrocnemius to the calcaneus (heel of the foot).

Right next to the Achilles we have the peroneus longus and brevis. These tendons are lateral and on the posterior side of the ankle bone. Then we have the cruciate ligament strapping all of these tendons together at the ankle.

All of these tendons can be sources of tendonitis. Of course, that's just an intense form of irritation that has happened over a long period of time. Keep doing the same thing that irritates it and you face worse problems. Forget the no pain, no gain theory.

Injuries to the Ankle

1.) Ankle sprain, lateral side ligaments
2.) Tibialis anterior strain to some of the extensors. This would hurt on the top of the foot.
3.) Achilles tendonitis
4.) Ankle strain medially
5.) Cruciate ligament and cruciate sprain.
6.) Flexor or plantar strain- Interosseous strain (between the metatarsals)
7.) Plantar fasciatis
8.) Posterior tibialis tendonitis
9.) And a combination of several strains together

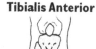

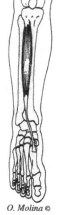

O. Molina ©

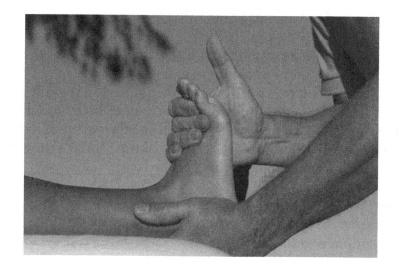

Tibialis Anterior and Tendonitis   test

This could come on gradually (tendonitis) or you can strain the tendon muscle complex on the top part of your arch. This is a common area for pain, but the pain could follow the whole tendon into the muscle. This can get injured from those company softball games, again. As we said, when you are not in good shape but you just push too hard these strains happen.

This is a common over training syndrome for runners, football players or basketball players. Sprinters and dancers get it occasionally, but not as often.

Putting your socks on can hurt, and any kind of flexion of the foot hurts. If walking hurts it means that you have tendonitis. Marathon running or jumping, and new hill training could fatigue this muscle. The muscle no longer supports the foot, and it makes the muscle over work, becoming stressed and eventually injured. Excess tension in the lower foot can cause this as well. I also believe improper warm ups play a large factor in long term problems with this muscle. No warm up at all (weekend warriors) leads to excess tension in the shin area (tibialis anterior- or often tibialis posterior), also causing "shin splints" down the road.

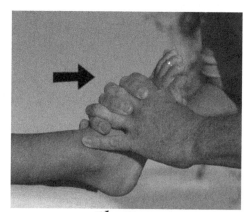

The Test

To test for this injury, with the patient prone, flex the foot (toes pointing towards face). The therapist then puts pressure on the dorsal aspect of the foot. (See picture above.) The pain could also be caused when you stand on your toes since you would be using your extensor muscle group.

These muscles are the extensor digitorum longus, the extensor hallucis longus, as well as the anterior tibialis

The Treatment

Of course DTF (deep transverse friction) and RICE are always indicated. Because this tendon is so readily available and the skin is right over the tendon with no fat layer in between, four or five treatments of DTF with the ice makes a big difference in the healing of the injury.

If it's from a long term over-use injury cycle, sometimes the massage is not as effective. It takes much more time to see results especially if there is lots of scar tissue present. A fast way to make progress here is with an injection of corticosteroid. It is a quick way to break the cycle. Then massage is much more effective after that. Remember, the athlete needs to lay off and rest. Swim, don't run.

When the foot is imbalanced, with flat feet or poor foundation, there is severe stress on the feet causing problems. For old injuries manipulations of the foot can create a really mobilizing effect by breaking up improperly formed scar tissue. Remember, it's all about balanced strength with the flexibility that is important for athletic excellence. Or, just pain free living for the normal, active person.

Ligaments of the ankle

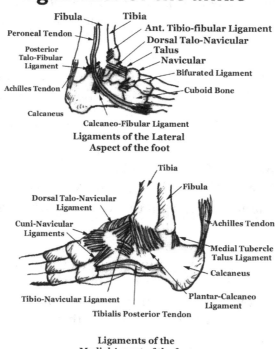

Fibula
Peroneal Tendon
Posterior Talo-Fibular Ligament
Achilles Tendon
Calcaneus
Tibia
Ant. Tibio-fibular Ligament
Dorsal Talo-Navicular
Talus
Navicular
Bifurated Ligament
Cuboid Bone
Calcaneo-Fibular Ligament

Ligaments of the Lateral Aspect of the foot

Tibia
Fibula
Dorsal Talo-Navicular Ligament
Cuni-Navicular Ligaments
Achilles Tendon
Medial Tubercle Talus Ligament
Calcaneus
Tibio-Navicular Ligament
Tibialis Posterior Tendon
Plantar-Calcaneo Ligament

Ligaments of the Medial Aspect of the foot

O. Molina ©

Ankle Sprain Lateral
(Outer part of the ligaments)

There aren't many athletes or active hikers that have not sprained an ankle. This is usually a fast move injury. It's the most common injury; about 90% of all injuries to the ankle are on these ligaments. In fact, in all sports and in daily life for that matter, it may be second only to the back injuries. It's often caused by weak arches (high arches or flat feet) and poor alignment of the bones in the feet, which make the torque move upwards. Also, from too much tension in the gastrocnemius (calf), which many athletes get by not stretching enough, or by improper base building. Remember, you can build muscle fast but the ligaments and the bones take longer to build. Yes, you can strengthen you ligaments and bones by applying the proper stress and resistance exercise program as you do for the muscles.

In a minor sprain maybe you overstretched the ligaments causing swelling and the tissue death (see chapter on sports traumas). Other times it's actually from tearing of the ligament fibers off the bone (the talo-fibular or calcaneo-fibular ligaments). Your ankle can really be unstable and it hurts to just put pressure or weight on the foot. That's usually how you know it's a ligament injury (see ligaments). Muscles and tendons will hurt with action. Bone fractures will hurt with everything. Ligaments will hurt with weight-bearing activities.

Running, jumping, landing wrong, getting hit in football, soccer, and rugby - all those quick turning sports can sprain an ankle. You may sometimes hear a pop! when sliding into a base or during a football or basketball game. It can swell real badly. If you don't know much about sports injuries it's scary to see for the first time. The problem is it creates tissue death and scar tissue if not properly treated. This creates a weak link in the area and it is primed for potential future injury.

I wish I knew in high school what I know now about sports medicine. It would have also been good if the coaches understood more about it, too. Once you have improperly formed scar tissue (IFST) it's more restricted and less flexible, as well as brittle and prone to re-injury. These injuries don't heal well and consequently are hurt at micro levels over and over again. The whole condition creates a cycle of pain, injury, tension, contraction, less movement, more injury, and pain. The swelling can get as big as a basketball in an acute injury.

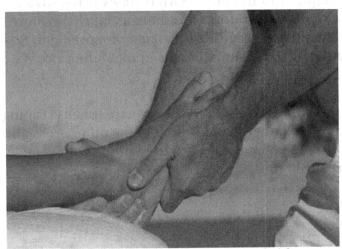

The Test: Put Pressure on Lateral Side

To test for the ligament the patient is prone and you flex the knee. You place one hand on the ankle itself and with the other hand; the therapist grabs the lower foot. You over extend the attachment of the ligaments, increasing the pull factor on the ligament and this will increase the pain. It's usually a very pinpointed, very specific and sharp pain. It can be very severe when it's an acute injury, so be careful. If it's a re-injury or it's an old and chronic injury it will still hurt but not as intensely. The level of pain is a good indication of the severity of the injury. Refer to a doctor if severe.

Treatment

The treatment for sprains is always RICE, even on the way to the doctor. It could heal up to one week faster for every hour you don't delay putting ice on it. We should know what that is by now; the ice with gentle movement will accelerate the healing cycle.

You can also increase the healing with DTF massage, and one of the best for old scar tissue is manipulation as well. Manipulation is not used in the acute state unless the bones of the feet are out of place. These moves can take great strength as well as knowledge and should only be done by a trained professional.

The two (DTF and manipulation) combined is, of course, the best way to improve the functioning of the area if it's an old, chronic, and second level rehab for an acute injury.

Some sports medicine doctors use injections of corticosteroid solution for these injuries. It takes great skill to get it to work, as you need to treat each individual tendon, ligament or fiber that is injured. If you just miss it, it's not very effective. They often times use the proliferant that helps tighten the area and stabilize imbalances. However, I have found the scar tissue, which makes it all too tight or rigid, is the problem more often.

Severe Tear on Ligaments

If the tear is severe then surgery may be indicated. Sometimes they sew the ligament back together or at worst staple it to the bone. Often times it requires a cast, although I have found that more and more doctors don't use them as much anymore. We have found that this creates too much scar tissue because of the lack of movement. So if a cast is required it should be followed with DTF and manipulations in rehabilitation. We need to increase or at least get back the flexibility in the joint.

Taping, however, is sometimes considered a better treatment. Taping the foot so that it's limited where you want it to be and has freedom in the other areas allows you to keep some mobility. When all of these technologies are used along with some exercise program and massage the results are the best.

Ankle Sprain Medially
(Ankle sprained inside)

The inside ankle sprain is much less common. This ligament on the inside part of the ankle is injured less frequently (tibio-talus and tibia-calcaneus). This could also be a ligamentous tear, as the deltoid or tibia talus ligament is fan shaped. It's more of a freak accident that causes this injury, while playing basketball or soccer, for example. For an old or chronic condition, this injury will happen more often to someone that is older at that company picnic, again, or one of those weekend warriors may sprain it in a running game. Most of us stiffen up with age, especially if you've pushed your body beyond what you had trained it to handle, and your ankles may be very tight.

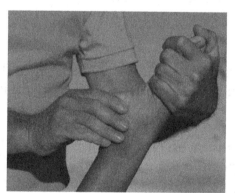
Test: Medial Tension Created

With patient prone or supine, take their heel in one hand and the ball of the foot with the other and twist increasing the space between the ligament attachments to stretch them. This, once again, should produce the same and very specific pain.

Treatment is the same as above, but for the best healing an arch support can take the pressure off the ligament. Remember, if it hurts to bear weight then it's a ligament. With an arch support the downward pressure will not strain the ligament and it will get better in time. Of course the DTF, injection, and orthodics will all help to heal the whole syndrome faster since this injury can be from a whole series of events, if it's not from a sudden impact or quick move.

Cruciate Ligament or Crural Sprain
(Ligament that straps the ankle)

Sometimes we have pain on the top of the foot or right around the ankle. It could be just about anywhere along this ligament that straps the ankle tendons together. It is one of the most common injuries in all sports. This injury usually comes from stepping wrong, twisting the foot and in sports where you cut too fast, sometimes from a hit to the foot from the side, as in football, rugby or soccer. Even baseball players get this injury. It is rarely from over use, unless we are talking about ballet dancers or professional modern dancers. This ligament holds all the tendons together similar to the one on your wrist. Of course if it's due to an impact, you can often times injure the tendons at the same time.

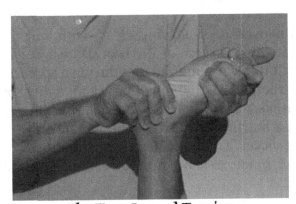
The Test: Lateral Tension

The test is to increase the strain on the ligament by bending the foot one way or the other. Then when you find the pain, palpation will give you further evidence.

Of course, the flexor muscle test should be done as well to see which hurts more: if its resistance, it's muscle /tendon and if it's the stretching or palpation then it's the ligament.

Treatment for ligaments is much the same -- DTF, RICE with some movement to prevent improper scar tissue formation (ISTF.) Plantar flexion and extension will aid in healing and keeping flexibility. Of course an injection can heal this faster sometimes and be very effective. The key in both treatments is to stay off of it; walking and even standing will irritate it further.

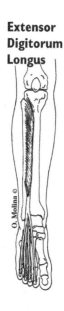

Extensor Digitorum Longus

O. Molina ©

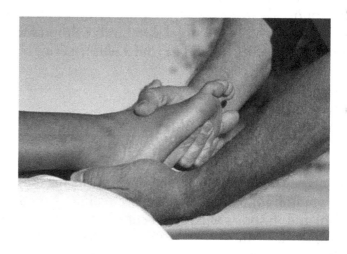

Midtarsal Strain
(Extensor Digitorum Longus) or tendonitis

This condition can be from over-use syndrome -- easy with long distance runners. It comes from weak arches and or an over stretch of the foot. Dance, football and soccer again are sources for these injuries. I thought one time that during a soccer game I had sprained that tendon. After walking or should I say limping home, I got a deep massage from my mom. It hurt like hell and I said it must be broken. Of course, after the next day when it was much worse, an x-ray revealed a hairline fracture of the metatarsals. I broke my foot all right, stepped in a hole playing soccer. To had to get a cast from the toes to just below the knee. Still I had been able to walk home, so make sure you evaluate the athlete carefully.

The Test

The test since it's tendo-muscular is to dorsiflex the foot and push down on the toes, just proximal to the toes. If it's a tendon it will hurt worse when doing it; if it's ligament just ROM (range of motion) will hurt.

This strain is mostly muscular or tendon, so the best treatment for both is RICE, DTF, some massage and mobilization to prevent improper scar tissue formation (ISTF). Once again, scar tissue is the culprit of re-injury. To prevent that, test for ligaments first and use DTF to accelerate the healing and prevent scar tissue.

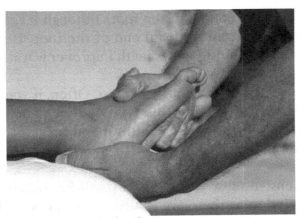
Pain in the Large Toe

The big toe strain is in this group of the foot injury. The muscle tendon here is the extensor hallucis longus. Kicking the soccer ball or football, in fact, almost any sport involving running can cause injuries here.

This injury can be confused with an anterior tibialis injury, so check carefully. Because the tendon runs into the big toe, when you test you need to be specific. It can come from over use in running but occurs more with dancers who point their foot, or ballet dancers who do intensive toe work. In fact, with most dancers and runners I spend a lot of time working on their feet, as this is a potential source of problems. Along with balancing the pelvis, they are our most focused areas of stress.

Feet need to be balanced as much as the pelvis. In fact, when I balance and work on the pelvis, I re-align the feet every time, as they will adjust and compensate with the weight distribution of the body.

The tests for the anterior tibialis, the extensor hallucis longus and the extensor digitorum longus are very close together, you just have to focus the pressure in slightly different areas for each muscle. (See pictures.)

The Test

Place your thumb right on the distal end of the first joint of the big toe and have the patient try and flex their big toe as you offer resistance. It could hurt anywhere from the first joint of the toe all the way up to the ankle if injured.

Treatment

The treatment will be the same for all of these tendons of the feet.

Flexor or Plantar Strain

This could be tendon (strain), or ligaments (sprain) or sometimes called an interosseous strain of the muscles that hold the joints of the toes together.

There will usually be pain in the bottom of the foot, although it can be on top just as easily. In fact, it can hurt all over the front or distal end of the foot. This is caused by excessive mileage in running, or from the cutting sports (with improper warm up or base building).

Maybe your running shoes don't offer enough support. Often, if you have flat feet this injury along with plantar fasciatis comes from this type of foot structure. Of course, you can prevent this by buying new shoes every few months if you run a lot. They support really well only for 50 miles or so nowadays.

Yeah! They are too expensive these days. We have all heard about Doctor Scholl's shoe inserts. They can help. Well, now there are really nice ones made by Nike. They are a bit expensive but they do last for a long time.

Building the base is most important in sports, like by running side to side, and for training not just straight ahead if that's what you do in the sport. I used to see all these football players and other athletes just running straight ahead, never doing heavy cuts. In basketball at least they made us go side to side in some training.

Anyway, we have learned a lot about athletic training since the fifties and sixties. As well as building up the tissue little by little, we also need to build the base and strengthen those ligaments. (See five laws of training). The last recourse if this doesn't work is to see a sports podiatrist and get some good orthodics.

Treatment: the same as above.

Plantar Muscles

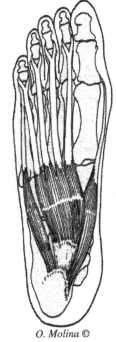

O. Molina ©

Plantar Fasciatis

(Injury to fascia at the bottom of the foot)

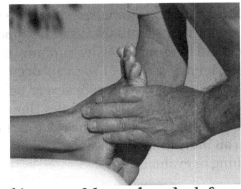

Push on top and bottom of the tendons, look for pain

Plantar fasciatis can be another pain on the bottom of the foot. It can also be felt more on the ball of the foot or the heel or on occasion in the arch. Its causes are over-use syndrome, of course, and by improper foot support, pushing the body before it was ready for the intensity, etc. What happens is the muscles under the foot can no longer create the support needed by the fascia. So with muscle fatigue the fascia starts to take the strain. Consequently it starts to tear because it's not as flexible nor designed to take that pressure like muscles can. It's not uncommon to have weekend warriors that run a marathon ending up with this injury. It also happens to fast-cutting sports athletes in an acute situation.

The worst part about this injury is that as soon as you feel it, which is usually in the morning, it hurts a little and then gets better and better as the day goes on, so you train again.

You injure the soft connective tissue which is trying to form on the bottom of the foot. These tear again and you are in a vicious cycle. Because the fascia has very little blood flow and is not very flexible, it suffers this re-injury problem. You must lay off completely for this to heal. Walking should be minimal, and it's very important to wear a heel lift or some good shoes during this time to take the pressure off the arch of the foot while the healing is occurring.

Remember, when you have an injury like this NO STRETCHING!!, no running, and certainly no jumping. You can have the athlete swim; they may even bike in the later stages of healing if it doesn't cause pain. But make sure they are not stretching the bottom of the foot when they bike or it will injure further. Of course the more you re-injure this area, the more scar tissue you form on it and the weaker it gets. Walking in sand is great for strengthening down the road, and if it's orthodics that are needed see a sports podiatrist.

They will fit you with the proper orthodics to prevent this problem in the future. Prevention is less painful than getting in the pain arena with it.

Posterior Tibialis Tendonitis
(Sometimes part of shin splints)

Posterior tibialis tendonitis is painful on the inner side and back of the ankle (tendon). It could also be associated with having shin splints injury at the same time along with the anterior tibialis since they are in the same muscle group.

They only differ by the location (see shin splints). Once again, flat feet or having the muscles doing extra work because of lack of arch support can contribute to this injury. If you get it gradually, it could be from excessive running, jumping sports or intense dancing. The tendon becomes very tender and swelling can occur and often gets worse after the particular activity. However, if it is a contact or severe twisting injury it can swell up like a balloon. I've seen ankles swell to three or four times their normal size. If you have someone with this level of injury, it's hard to determine the exact injury. Sometimes asking the right questions will give you an indication of how it happened. We always do this first with injuries, anyway, before touching or evaluating.

The Test

The test for this injury is opposite to the test of the peroneus group. The patient is supine and you take their knee and bend it, slightly supporting the knee, then you push on the metatarsals or the side of the foot laterally stressing the tendon. They push the foot medially with some dorsiflexion and you offer the resistance. Caution: When you have a very swollen patient, it may better to wait until after RICE.

For tendonitis it can be misleading, because once the athlete warms up, the pain is better. It's like the Achilles tendonitis, you get into the vicious cycle and keep training and it keeps getting worse. The pain is usually worse in the morning. You need to stop the activity at least until it stops hurting at rest, and then gradually build later.

Treatment: same as above.

Peroneus Longus

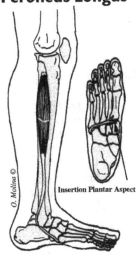

O. Molina ©

Insertion Plantar Aspect

Peroneus Tendonitis

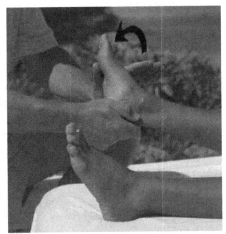

Test

(Pain on the latter side of the ankle)

Peroneus longus and brevis are the two stabilizing muscles of the ankle. They also help lift the leg in walking and running with a slight pull to the outside of the foot (lateral dorsiflexion). These tendons are also supported by the cruciate ligament on the back side of the foot. There is often irritation in this area due to athletes not stretching enough or warming up their lower legs or calf's (actually the gastrocnemius) but that is a good stretch for the peroneus as well. The athletes who are most commonly injured are rugby players because they tend to stretch very little and are the epitome of weekend warriors. "If it hurts, drink more beer!" This injury can come from the same situations as with the posterior tibialis -- cutting sports, twisting ankles or professional dancers can overwork the area. Once again, weak arches, may be a contributing factor, or exaggerated pronation (toes turned in)can stress these tendons.

The Test

To test the peroneus, lay the patient supine and have them straighten the leg with your hand on the heel and the other hand on the lateral side of the foot. Have them push their foot outwards in external rotation (lateral). The therapist offers resistance pushing medially, which should cause the pain in the area that's injured. Treatment is the same as above: RICE, DTF, and if the conditions are chronic, we know that injections are a great way to treat this injury.

Posterior Muscles

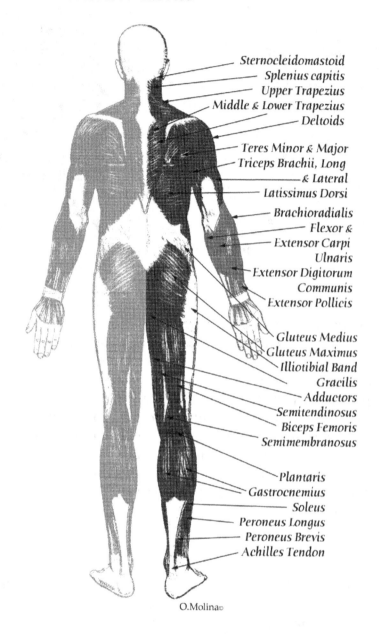

Sternocleidomastoid
Splenius capitis
Upper Trapezius
Middle & Lower Trapezius
Deltoids

Teres Minor & Major
Triceps Brachii, Long
& Lateral
Latissimus Dorsi

Brachioradialis
Flexor &
Extensor Carpi
Ulnaris
Extensor Digitorum
Communis
Extensor Pollicis

Gluteus Medius
Gluteus Maximus
Illiotibial Band
Gracilis
Adductors
Semitendinosus
Biceps Femoris
Semimembranosus

Plantaris
Gastrocnemius
Soleus
Peroneus Longus
Peroneus Brevis
Achilles Tendon

O.Molina©

The end

References and Recommended Books

James Cyriax, M.D., *Orthopedic Medicine, Volume I, II*, Wilkins CO, Baltimore MD, 1977

Paul Vinger, M.D., *Sports Injuries*, PSG Publishing, Littleton MA, 1981

Stanley Hopperfield, *Physical Examination of the Spine and Extremities.*

Ben Benjamin Ph.D., *Listen to Your Pain*, Penguin Books, 1984.

Gabe Mirkin, M.D. and Marshall Hoffman, Little, Brown and Company, 1978.

My friend and great athlete, Terry Albriton, Honolulu, Hawaii, 1978.

Jack Meager, *Sports Massage*, Dolphin Books, New York, NY 1980.

Ken Dychtwald, *Body Mind*, Published in Britain, Wildwood House, 1978

James Fixx, *The Complete Book of Running*, Random House, NY, 1977.

Manual of Structural Kinesiology by Thompson.

M. Hungaford Ph.D., *Sport massage workshops and writing*

Richard Phaye, Sports massage expert from Eugene, Oregon.

Other sources: Dr. James F. Balch, Phyllis A. Balch, C.N.C., and Dr. Richard Podell, and Dr. Anrew Weil.

Many, many other books……stay in touch see my web site…

www.molinamassage.com   www.yourbeautifulbody.org

coming soon "Better back book"   see at www.betterbackbook.com

Printed in the United States
By Bookmasters